PALEO

The Healthy New You with Paleo

(Includes All-time Best Paleo Recipes -- Breakfast,
Lunch, Dinner & Desserts)

Annabel Jacobs

Amazon Kindle 2016 Edition

PALEO

The Healthy New You with Paleo

(Includes All-time Best Paleo Recipes -- Breakfast, Lunch, Dinner & Desserts)

Introduction

BREAKFAST

Paleo Garlic Breadsticks (Just Don't Eat Them All Yourself)

Eggplant Bolognese with Zucchini Noodles (Low Carb)

LUNCH

Easy Paleo Shepherd's Pie

Meatball Zucchini Skillet

Paleo Pulled Pork Sliders

Crock-Pot Roast

Tuna Avocado Lettuce Wraps (Makes the Perfect Lunch)

Finger Lickin' Chipotle Meatballs

Fennel and Brussels Sprouts Sirloin Rolls

Easy Paleo Spaghetti Squash & Meatballs

Paleo Crock Pot Cashew Chicken

Spicy Slow Cooker Chorizo Chili

Perfect Tomatillo Salsa Verde

Homemade Herbed Paleo Mayonnaise

Homemade Paleo Ketchup with a Kick

Homemade Paleo Honey Mustard from Scratch

Melt In Your Mouth Slow Cooker Beef Brisket

Bacon-Wrapped Roasted Asparagus

Simple Cod Piccata

Paleo BLT Frittata

Spaghetti Squash Shrimp Scampi (Grain-Free & Low Carb)

Honey Balsamic Roasted Brussels Sprouts

Paleo Shrimp Fried "Rice"

Sausage and Kale "Pasta" Casserole

Basic Balsamic Steak Marinade

Rosemary Beets with Garlicky Kale

Kale and Red Pepper Frittata

Paleo Chocolate Cookies (I Can't Get Enough of These)

Paleo French Toast with Blueberry Syrup

Lavender Maca Brownies (Dairy & Grain Free)

Green Kale Smoothie with Mango

Easy Paleo Shepherd's Pie

Spicy Avocado Dill Dressing

No-Bake Walnut Cookies (Grain-Free & Gluten-Free)

Stove-top "Cheesy" Paleo Chicken Casserole

Legendary Gluten-Free Blueberry Crisp (YUM!)

Paleo Chicken Tortilla Soup

Butternut Squash & Kale Beef Stew

Bacon and Tomato Quiche

DINNER

Prosciutto-Wrapped Berries

Almond Joy Sunday

Spiced Autumn Apples Baked in Brandy

Curried Paleo Cauliflower Soup

Fresh and Easy Arugula Pesto

Homemade Paleo BBQ Sauce (YUM)

Basil Pesto

Radicchio Pesto

Dill & Lemon Baked Salmon in Parchment

Healthy Low Carb Crustless Quiche Recipe

Sun-Dried Tomato Quiche

Asparagus Quiche with Spaghetti Squash Crust

Coconut Crust Quiche

Garden Pea, Feta & Mint Tart

Garlicky Collard Pie

Crustless Broccoli and Sausage Quiche

Crustless Mini Quiches

Broccoli Egg Bake (So Wholesome & Healthy)

Meatball Sandwich with Zucchini "Bread" & Coconut Curry Sauce

Zucchini "bread" and coconut sauce

Vegetarian Thai Red Curry with Squash

Paleo Cauliflower "Rice"

Simple Beef and Broccoli Stir Fry

Homemade Sweet and Salty Paleo Granola

Easy Paleo Slow Cooker Pot Roast

Hearty Paleo Jambalaya (Try This!)

Shrimp & Grits (Paleo Style)

Paleo Turkey Pesto Meatballs

DESSERTS

Paleo Antioxidant Berry Shake

Balsamic Green Bean Salad

Chocolate Bavarian Cheesecake

Raw Brownie Bites

Faux Paleo Napoleon

Homemade Strawberry Fruit Leather

Paleo Coconut Cupcakes with Chocolate Frosting

Easy Homemade Gluten-Free Energy Bars

Coconut Macaroons with Chocolate and Pistachio

The Best Paleo Brownies (Chocolaty Goodness)

Homemade Baked Cinnamon Apple Chips

Introduction

I want to thank you and congratulate you for downloading the book, *"PALEO: The Healthy New You with Paleo (Includes All-time Best Paleo Recipes -- Breakfast, Lunch, Dinner & Desserts)"*.

This book contains best recipes, proven steps and strategies on how you can enjoy the healthy benefits of eating on Paleo diet.

For years, many Americans are considered either overweight or obese. The rapidly increasing obesity rate is also becoming a problem. Because of these, different kind of diets and weight loss tips were introduced. Fad diets encouraged many Americans to stay healthy and fit. One of those diets is Paleo Diet.

Paleo diet is also referred as the "Caveman Diet". It emphasize that eating vegetables, fruits and other whole foods is the simplest way to live a longer life. Early humans consumed and thrived on foods naturally found in their environment, and wild animals that eat grass and living organisms. Many scientists deemed that this is the main reason why our ancestors were energized, physically fit and healthy. This book may show how you can have the energy, physique and health similar to a caveman.

There are chapters that explain the basics of Paleo diet, its origin and its potential benefits. Experiments and studies performed on the diet is also included, which identify the specific benefits of the diet regimen to people with high blood sugar levels, Type 2 diabetes and obese.

By flipping the pages of this book, you will find out different tips that can help you sustain with the meal plan. It can guide you in making your own Paleo diet plan for a week. For a starter, you can use the sample of 7 day meal plan found in this book. That way, your easy and healthy transition to Paleo lifestyle is guaranteed.

Thanks again for downloading this book, I hope you enjoy it!

Chapter 1

Paleo Diet 101

When the word diet comes to mind, many people assume that its only purpose is weight loss. Weight loss encourages many of us to try different diets that had been introduced for the past several years.

There are diets that focus on eating vegetables and fruits such as vegetarian diet, Vegan diet that stay away from dairy and other animal product, and Gluten-free diet that encourage people to refrain from eating foods containing gluten.

Each diet has a different approach in helping us to lose weight. However, those diets can make our body healthier because it can help us prevent certain diseases and food allergies, and can keep our body healthy and fit. Diet regimen can improve body function, emotional and mental health. You are able to get these benefits from Paleo diet.

What is Paleo Diet?

Also known as "The Caveman Diet", Paleo diet is a traditional but modern diet regimen that emulates the healthy eating of the cave mans during the Paleolithic era. It focuses on consuming wild plants and animals eaten by humans. Paleo diet advocates recommend that you should stay away from any foods that were not available to humans at the time of the Paleolithic era. These foods are dairy products, processed oils, legumes and refined sugar.

The "Caveman Diet" may sound like a weird fad diet to you, but in fact, it is not. Back in the days wherein civilization, processed foods and development are inexistent, humans are accustomed on eating real, whole unprocessed foods. Those foods are healthier and harmless to our bodies. According to sources, humans have adapted best to whole foods such as meat, plants and seafood over the past 200,000 years.

However, when the agriculture came on the scene nearly 10,000 years ago, humans did not have enough time to completely adapt on eating modern foods such as sugar, wheat and chemically processed seed oils and vegetables. Many supporters of Paleo diet believed that this is one of the reasons why many people suffered cardiovascular diseases, autoimmune disorders, type 2 diabetes and obesity. They claimed that industrialized food might be the primary cause of such diseases. That's why the Paleo diet encourages you to return to more ancestral way of eating in order to prevent and fight those illnesses.

Chapter 2

Paleo Diet, and its Rich and Healthy History

Just like any other popular fad diets, Paleo diet has a rich history. For a starter, the Caveman Diet includes healthy foods such as vegetables that only "cavemen" would have had access to, and animals fed by grass. The following information may demonstrate why eating figs, green leafy vegetables and naturally grown fruits would be best for us.

The history of Paleolithic diet was traced back from our ancestors, the Apes. Many researchers believed that the ape began to live on the planet around 50 million years ago. It was claimed that early primates had the same dietary habits of the current primate species such as chimps and bonobos. That diet was likely composed of leaves, gums, fruits and stalks. They also consumed eggs, insects and small animals.

Apes ate protein-rich foods. Unlike the protein eaten by modern humans, these primates ate protein that comes from plants. Modern proteins are incomplete proteins that do not have all the nutrients needed for life. Our ape ancestor's plant protein intake is similar to the recommended protein dietary intake of today. Vegetables and plants supply fiber, which is much better than the fiber found in simple carbohydrates of processed foods.

Vitamins and minerals intake of primate are also higher because they ate plant material. Their diet during that era consisted of little to no salt. Their cholesterol and fat intake are much lower as well.

The diet of early primates may show why it makes sense to eat a diet composed of foods that we have the adapted the ability to digest.

Considering that they got used to eating vegetables, and animals fed naturally, their diet is high in fiber that keeps them healthy.

Here comes the Paleolithic Age

There are different theories claiming that our ancestors left their homes in the forest during the Paleolithic era. Some researchers speculated that the growth of their population or geographical changes urged the early humans to migrate and travel longer distances to look for food. Evidence suggests that as our ancestors entered evolution, they went from being scavengers to a forager. Based on the dental records gathered by several scientists, it is likely that this change was due to the inclusion of animal flesh or meat to their diet. They eventually learn to fish and hunt, which supply healthy fat to the brain resulting in brain development.

Around 2.5 million years ago, evidence illustrates that animal meat earned its big role in our ancestors' diet. It has been found that early humans have experienced changes in the shape of their incisors, reduced in molar size, and less cranial robusticy of their teeth. Scientists pointed out that these changes definitely occur from tearing or grinding meat. They also believed that the inclusion of meat in their diet is responsible for the evolution the early humans to Australopithecines to the more recognizable species known as Homo Erectus. Because meat supplies them with healthy fats, they are able to use tools when hunting. As our ancestors continue on eating healthy fats, their brains keep on to developing as well, enabling them to have interaction skills, and abilities to make plans and tools.

For this reason, the supply of fiber and other phytochemicals to early humans were reduced. Although the inclusion of meat in the diet ultimately led to brain development for humans, it is believed that the toxic chemicals found in meat such as "cyanogenic glycosides" cause a disruption in the intestinal tract. Cyanogenic glycosides are also found in grain.

Then Comes the Neolithic Era

Our ancestors discovered the grains, one of the sources of bread, rice and other carbohydrates foods. They found that grains can be stored and used in case of food shortage. However, grains should be cooked to make it indigestible, making it not ideal for food source. The growth population during the Neolithic Era makes grain foods as the most attractive alternative food source to feed a small civilization, and eventually making it the major food source.

The growing consumption of grain led to less vegetables and fruits intake. Because of those changes, vitamins and minerals that are needed by the body decreases as well. Consuming less fruits and vegetables is disadvantageous to the body. It can prevent the body from obtaining nutrients needed in fighting certain diseases like cancer.

Paleo Diet During the Industrial Era

The industrial era influenced the diet of our ancestors. It makes them forget all about the natural-growth foods that are healthier and harmful to our body. Aside from the fact that carbohydrates became one of the main food sources, humans started to consume sugar cane and alcohol. The creation of vegetable oils also put an imbalance in the omega 3-6 ratio of the body. As time went by, different processed foods were also created. The beef industry benefitted from unhealthy cows. They were able to gathered mass amount of meat, including unhealthy fats from those cows, by feeding them animal grain foods and hormones instead of grass food. Animal grain foods created larger fat stores and tastier meat, which are more advantageous to their businesses. Cows that have an unhealthy diet are deprived from omega 3 content found on grass.

What the Paleo Diet's History is Pointing Out

Humans are the only primates that include grains as a major staple in their diet. Because of this, vegetables that are healthier and harmful to our body are being excluded. It is proven that phytochemicals can fight different types of cancer in the body.

On the contrary, grains can only fight one type of cancer, and causes insulin resistance that can lead to many health complications like Type 2 diabetes and high blood pressure. These are the reasons why we need to replace grains with vegetables and fruits on our diet. Doing so does not mean we should completely avoid grains, Paleo diet emphasizes that we should not make grain foods as the staple in our diet.

Chapter 3

What Science Says About Paleo?

You may think that the previous paragraphs you have read on this article were all claims without evidence. While the history of Paleo Diet might not be enough to prove its healthy benefits, several studies have been made to determine if it really does works.

The Paleo diet imitate the diet of our hunter-gatherer ancestors who lived longer years. According to its rich history, early humans are healthier than the modern ones because their diets are based on natural foods such as vegetables, fruits and unprocessed meat. Paleo diet also suggests that processed foods such as dairy, sugar and grains should be avoided.

The following studies may illustrate the good effects of Paleo diet to humans.

- According to a 2008 study called the "Effects of a Short-term Intervention with Paleolithic diet in Healthy Volunteers", humans can experience weight loss by using the Caveman diet. The study examined 14 healthy medical students, 5 males and 9 females, respectively. They were instructed to undergo a paleo diet for three weeks. No control group is included in this study.

  Three weeks later, the participants lose 2.3 kgs or 5 lbs. Their body mass index was reduced by 0.8 and their waist circumference decreased by 1.5 cm (0.6 inches).The participants' systolic blood pressure also went down.

  Therefore, the researchers concluded that the individuals who used Paleo diet experienced significant weight loss and had a mild reduction in their systolic blood pressure and waist circumference.

- In 2009 study called Beneficial effects of a Paleolithic Diet on Cardiovascular Risk Factors in Type 2 Diabetes: a Randomized Cross-

Over Pilot Study", the paleo diet can caused improve cardiovascular risk factors and more weight loss, in comparison to the Diabetes diet.

The cross-over study involved 13 patients suffering from Type 2 Diabetes. The 10 men and 3 women were instructed to eat a Paleo diet composed of fish, fruits, lean meat, vegetables, root vegetables, eggs and nuts. They also ate in a Diabetes diet that is created in accordance with the dietary guidelines for two consecutive 3-month periods. The researchers analyzed the participants' weight, waist circumference, serum lipids, blood pressure, glycated haemoglobin and C-reaction protein. Their dietary intake was evaluated by using a 4-day weighed food records.

Three months later, the participants lost 3 kgs of more weight. Their waistlines lost 4 cm more, compared to their weight loss in a Diabetes diet. The study participants ' HbA1c, a marker for 3-month blood sugar levels, were reduced y 0.4 percent more while they are on Paleo diet. Their HDL rose by 3 mg. on the Caveman diet regimen than the Diabetes diet, and their triglycerides went down as well.

The study concluded that Paleo diet can cause significant improvements iin cardiovascular risk factors and can results in more weight loss that the Diabetes diet.

- The third study that evaluated Paleo Diet is called "A Paleolithic diet improves glucose tolerance more than a Mideterranean-like diet in individuals with ischaemic heart disease", which was reported n 2007. Twenty nine men suffering from heart disease and with elevated blood sugars or type 2 diabetes have participated in the study. The researchers divided them into two groups. One group followed the Mediterranean—like diet while the other eats in accordance with the Paleolithic diet. Neither of the group was restricted from calories.

Researchers measured the participants' gluten intolerance, weight, insulin levels and waist circumference for 12 weeks. The glucose tolerance test is used to determine how quickly glucose is cleared from the blood. The test is considered as a marker for a person's insulin resistance and diabetes risk.

- According to a 2009 study called "Metabolic and physiologic improvements from consuming a Paleolithic, hunter-gatherer type diet", Paleo diet can reduce an individual's insulin level, diastolic blood pressure, triglycerides, total cholesterol and LDL cholesterol.

The researchers performed a metabolically, outpatient and controlled study among nine non-obese sedentary healthy volunteers. During the study period, they put the volunteer's findings when they were on their usual diet in comparison to the time when they ate in a Paleolithic diet. The volunteers consumed their usual diet during 3 days. Three-ramp up diets associated with increased in potassium and fiber for 7 days was instructed. After that, they underwent the Paleolithic-type of diet for 7 days.

The participants' total cholesterol was reduced by 16 percent, their LDL cholesterol was decreased by 22 percent, triglycerides went down by 35 percent and insulin AUC was reduced by 39 percent.

- In a study released on 2013, it indicated the possible benefits of Paleo diet to weight loss. The study was called "A Paleolithic-type diet causes strong tissue-specific effects on ectopic fat deposition in obese postmenopausal women".

The study authors observed 10 healthy women with BMI over 27 who have consumed a modified Paleo diet for 5 weeks. After the study period, the female participants' blood pressure decreased from an average of 125/82 mmHG to 115/75 mmHg. Their fasting blood sugars reduced by 6.35 mg/dL (0.35 mmol/L) and fasting insulin levels were decreased by 19 percent. The women's total cholesterol reduced by 33 mg/dl (0.85 mmol/L).

It was concluded that the women had major reductions in liver fat and lost weight during the 5 week trial. They also experienced some health improvements.

These studies cannot make any conclusions regarding the effectiveness and benefits of a Paleo diet. However, the scientific findings of the 5 studies were promising.

Chapter 4

What a Paleo Diet Can Do For You?

In case the scientific studies are not enough to prove the benefits of Paleo diet, here is the list of the healthy advantages of the Caveman diet to your life.

If you think that you need to starve yourself for 40 days and 40 nights in Paleo, you better think again. Paleolithic diet does not encourage you to stop eating. The diet regimen will teach you how to eat healthier foods. The problem with Americans' diet nowadays is they think that their body is invincible, making them eat processed foods, sugars and unhealthy fats that can be harmful to the body. With Paleo diet, a person just has to eat in a similar fashion as a caveman. Doing so may help them obtain the following benefits.

Paleo diet provides you with healthy cells

Every cell in our body is made of both saturated and unsaturated fats. The cells rely upon the healthy balance of the two so that the body can function properly. Fortunately, the paleo diet can naturally provide the balance of fats because it advised people to consume meats that have healthy fats. The diet regimen suggests healthy amount of fats in the body unlike other fad diets that limit one or another.

It provides you with more muscle, but less fat

Animal flesh is recommended in paleo diet. This type of meat comes with a healthy protein that is very anabolic, which is good for building new muscle cells. More muscle cells in the body are good for metabolism, keeping an individual's body fit. The muscles need energy to move. To be able to move, bigger muscles should store energy in them to permit the body to provide energy to the muscle cells and not to the fat cells.

Through a healthy paleo diet, the body will have more muscle cells than fat cells. Due to this, any extra energy will be moved to glycogen in the muscles, preventing the triglycerides. On the other hand, the fat cells will obtain triglycerides.

Gives you all Vitamins and Minerals

A large part of Paleo diet is consists of vegetables and fruits. The diet plan recommended that people should eat variety of veggies depending on seasons. Because of these, people eating a Paleo diet obtain the right vitamins and minerals needed by their body.

Keeps your brain healthy

Cold water fish is considered the best sources of protein and fat that are good for the brain. For example, a salmon fat is packed with omega 3 fatty acids, a nutrient that is lacking from the American diet. Omega 3 fatty acids contain DHA, which is good for the heart, eyes and brain development. Therefore, lack of omega 3 fatty acids can prevent the brain from developing and functioning properly. Fortunately, Cold water fish like Salmon is recommended in the Caveman diet.

Have More Energy with Paleo Diet

A typical American breakfast is made of a sugar coffee match with a bagel with a cream cheese of muffin. This kind of breakfast is considered harmful for the body because of its amount of sugar and fats. It can eventually results in type 2 diabetes and insulin resistance.

Paleo diet is different, however. It helps a person strategically choose foods that are healthy and can prevent diseases.

Caveman diet increased insulin sensitivity.

When a person consumes sugar on a regular basis, it is likely that the body will desensitize itself from sugary foods, such as ice cream and pastries because it has the ability to reject unnecessary nutrients. The human body only needs an appropriate amount of energy, and it creates a certain threshold or limitation on its ability to store energy. When that threshold is reach, the cells will automatically reject more energy, turning it into fat instead. If the condition continues, the body will likely develop an insulin sensitivity, which may prevent you from recognizing whether you are full or not.

However, eating on a Paleo diet improves the blood pressure and glucose tolerance of an individual. It also decreases insulin secretion, raise insulin sensitivity and improves lipid profiles.

Limiting Fructose

The Caveman diet considered that the body digests fructose differently than carbohydrates. This is the reason why the diet regimen recommends limiting the amount of fructose intake of the body. It suggests that dieters should choose the perfect fruit while eating on a Paleo diet. For example, it may be better to choose kiwi over banana because kiwi contains more Vitamin C. At least 2-3 pieces of fruits are the recommended fruit intake in this diet.

Improves Digestion and Absorption

The paleo diet suggests that people should foods that they have the ability to digest over thousands of years. This means that our eating habit should be similar to cave man, in which they consumed meat from animals who ate grass and vegetables free from chemicals.

There is no question whether or not people can tolerate starch or grass-fed beef. It is evident that our ancestors survived and thrived off those natural processed foods. Because of this, many researchers believed that Paleo diet can improve one's digestion and absorption of nutrients. It may also cure digestion problems.

Limit food allergies

Some people do not have the ability to digest seeds, dairy and other products. Because of this, people suffering from food allergies may benefit from Paleo diet. Paleo diet recommends to lessen foods that are known to be allergens for most people. The diet regimen advises to minimize the amount of grains, wheat and other foods that are not consumed by our early ancestors during the Paleolithic era. In a Paleo diet, you can occasionally consume those foods and not entirely avoid it.

This diet may provide many fibers to the body. With adequate water intake and smaller intake of sodium, Paleo diet can reduce the bloat that many people experience on a Western diet. It also mend the gut flora, which is significant in maintaining a healthy digestion.

Paleo can sustain your weight loss

You can experience significant weight loss while eating on a paleo diet. The caveman diet improves your metabolism, digestion and gut health, it can eventually to weight loss. The diet regimen is also design as a low-carb diet. Given that low-carb diet maintains an appropriate of carb intake but not avoiding it entirely, it may help you lose weight. By limiting the carbohydrate intake, you may avoid unwanted fat gain, which is usually caused by excessive carbs.

The paleo diet is also focus on maintaining a healthy ratio of omega 3- fatty acids, which assist our body in burning stored body fat. With this, you can enjoy an active lifestyle; have a stress management and better sleep.

Beat Hyperglycemia

People suffering from acute or chronic hyperglycemia experience symptoms of hungry and angry, which is usually called "hangry". This condition also occurs when the blood sugar went down and an individual gets hungry associated with fatigue, disorientation, irritability and foggy mind.

Meals made of protein and fat are satisfying, which is recommended in Paleo diet. The energy produced by fat, protein and some glucose can be released slowly and evenly throughout the day. Because of this, the blood sugar levels of an individual may become stable. This also allows the body to be energized throughout the day. Therefore, the body will experience less hunger and prevents crazy mood swings.

Chapter 5

Starting the Paleo Way of Eating

It has been reported that Paleo diet has many benefits. Those benefits are supported by studies and experiments conducted regarding the Caveman diet. While its good effects may not be guaranteed, the diet regimen may actually work because it is concentrated on real foods instead of processed foods and refined sugars. A nutritionist stated that real foods contain the right portions of nutrients that will help a person maintain blood sugar and keep their hunger hormones stable.

Typically, the basic guidelines for starting a Paleo diet are associated with skipping grains, packaged snacks, dairy, legumes and sugar. The paleo eating habit is focused on vegetables, fruit, meat, eggs, seafood, nuts, fats and oils. Doing so may seem easy but it requires determination, discipline and perseverance from someone to be successful on Paleo diet.

The following guidelines would be helpful in beginning your Paleo diet lifestyle.

Clean out the Kitchen

Your kitchen says everything about your diet and eating habits. For this reason, it is important to start to make changes on your kitchen if you want to eat on a cave man diet.

Gather all the foods that should avoid in Paleo diet. These foods are grains, cereal, vegetable oils,beans,, yogurt , cheese and milk. Get it and toss them in the trash or donate it for goodwill. This is what you should do if you want to avoid temptation and stick on your diet regimen.

You can also choose the baby-step way. You can cut out dairy products during your first week, and then eliminate refined grains for the second week. On the third week, you can skip all grains and so on until you are able to follow the Paleo diet. Choosing the baby step may help your body gradually adjust with the diet plan, reducing cravings and other withdrawal symptoms.

Concentrate on your Motivation

Many people turn into the cave man diet in order to improve their medical problems, such as gastrointestinal disorders, allergies and autoimmune conditions. Some people used Paleo diet to feel better everyday because they believe the plan is the healthiest way to eat. No matter what reason you have to start the Paleo regimen, your reason will help you stick with the guidelines and be meticulous about what you eat. Concentrate on your motivation, follow the guidelines no matter how strict it is and enjoy the healthy benefits of Paleo diet.

Follow the 85/15 Rule

After the first months of following the Paleo basic guidelines, many experts suggested the 85/15 rule. The 85/15 approach means that 85 percent of your time should be spend on eating on caveman diet while the remaining

15 percent should be the time you can eat non-paleo foods such as hamburger, granola bar or cookout.

During this period, you need to pay attention to the reaction of your body on the approach. For example, if you ate a scoop of ice cream and woke up feeling bloated the next day, you should decide if that discomfort is worthy in the future.

Try Cooking

Paleo diet is based on whole and fresh foods. Due to this, it is easier for people to make your home cook meals rather than order take out from restaurants. It would be difficult for you to determine the ingredients used in meals cooked in restaurants, especially fast food chains.

However, cooking your own meals, in accordance with the guidelines inn Paleo diet, may be a good opportunity for you to experiment on new foods. It may be a challenged to buy the weirdest looking vegetables in the supermarket and turn it into a delicious meal.

Expect a Setback

People eating on Paleo diet have their share of setbacks. It is given that you might experience a few withdrawals or slip back into your normal eating habits. Under such circumstances, it may helpful to surround yourself with people that gone through the same thing, such as support groups of Paleo diet. Interacting with people who understand your motivation, and the benefits of the caveman diet would help you transition with your new healthy lifestyle easily.

Learn to Decode the labels

Decoding the labels would be helpful when shopping for Paleo diet. You already know that you need to skip cookies, doughnuts, and crackers. However, there are other foods that are also not advisable for Paleo such as peanut butter, dried fruits with added sugars, soy sauce, malt vinegars, lunch meats and marinade sauces. You should be mindful of the ingredients listed on labels when choosing your Paleo foods.

Make an Oil Change

Instead of using canola, corn or soybean oil for sautéing, use coconut oil or lard when cooking your Paleo meals. High-quality saturated oils such as coconut oil and lard are healthy for cooking because it is more stable and will not oxidize when heated. Oxidation may release damaging free radicals, which occurs when vegetable oils such as canola or corn, are heated on a pan.

When it comes to lard, animal fats from grass fed cows contains more omega-3 fatty acids and conjugated linoleic acid that may help that body's fat burning process. Butter from grass-fed cows is also recommended by experts. You can also use avocado oil, olive oil and walnut oil for cold applications.

Chapter 6

What to Eat and What Not to Eat on Paleo

The Paleo diet is designed to teach you about how to eat like a cave man. Meaning, you can only eat foods that our early ancestors thrived and survived on during the Paleolithic era. These foods do not include dairy products, some carbohydrates and other processed goods.

To be able to specify which foods are allowed and not allowed on a Paleo diet, a compilation of the two categories are listed below. This framework may help you determine what you can eat and not eat on the diet regimen,

What to Eat on Paleo Diet

Vegetables

You can eat all kinds of vegetables on Paleo diet, including sweet potatoes. Experts recommended that organic veggies are better because it is free from pesticides that come from chemicals. It was suggested that vegetables that has the less transit time between the farm and consumer is healthier because more nutrients are retained.

- Asparagus
- Artichoke
- Beets
- Broccoli
- Brussels Sprouts
- Cabbage
- Carrots
- Cauliflower
- Celery
- Collard Greens
- Cucumber
- Eggplant
- Endive
- GreenOnions
- Kale
- Mushrooms
- Mustard Greens

Fruits

Generally, the Paleo diet rule that applies on vegetables is the same when it comes to fruits. Fruits produced locally and organic are better compared to fruits imported from other country, and those that are sprayed with chemicals and pesticides.

If you are really trying to lose weight but are not as active at all, it may be helpful if you limit your fruit intake. One or two pieces of fruits a day will do, because the nutrients and sugar some fruits contain may add up to the carbs.

- Apple
- Apricot
- Avocado
- Banana
- Blackberries
- Blueberries
- Boysenberries
- Cantaloupe
- Cherimoya
- Cherries
- Cranberries
- Figs
- Grapefruit
- Grapes
- Guava
- Honeydew
- Kiwi
- Lemon
- Lime
- Lychee
- Mango
- Orange
- Papaya
- Passion Fruit
- Peaches
- Pears
- Persimmon
- Pineapple
- Plums
- Pomegranate
- Raspberries
- Star Fruit
- Strawberries

- Tangerine
- Watermelon

Meats and Eggs

Considerably, you can eat meats and eggs freely. When it comes to Paleo diet, however, it is advised that you should eat meat products from animals that were raised in pasture and grass fed. Dieters should also steer clear from meats produced with preservatives, additional flavourings such as a nitrates.

- Beef - Make sure that it is locally produced. Limit your beef intake, otherwise.

- Buffalo/Bison – A healthy alternative for beef because the buffalo industry is not as widespread as the beef industry. This means that there is a less chance that the meat is grass-fed and raised in pastures.

- Chicken –Enjoy all parts of chicken, ranging from breast, legs, thigh and wings. Chicken breast is a great source of protein and may serve as a staple food for Paleo dieters.

- Eggs – You can eat all types of eggs on the Caveman diet. It is a source of food back of our ancestors during the Paleolithic Era. Choose for eggs that are cage-free and organic variety.

- Lamb – You can make lamb as your regular meat option. Although it contains more fats than other meats, it is a good source of protein for Paleo dieters.

- Pork – Choose pork meats that are more organic and chemical free, unlike pork cuts you can find on supermarket.

- Turkey – another poultry option would be turkey. You can but it on many supermarkets and grocery stores, but be sure to opt roasted turkey breast over cold cuts that has nitrates and sodium.

Seafood –All species of fish and seafood are fine. Just be mindful of the mercury levels and ecological practices used to obtain or catch those resources. Know that smaller fish typically has the less bio-accumulation of toxins and heavy metals but it has high levels of omega 3 fatty acids.

- Bass
- Clams
- Halibut
- Lobster
- Mackerel
- Salmon
- Sardines
- Swordfish
- Tilapia
- Trout
- Tuna

Fats, Nuts and Seeds

The good thing about Paleo diet is that healthy fats plays an important role in balancing the amount of nutrients obtains by your body. All kinds of nuts are good. The same goes to seeds. When it comes to oils, go for a non-vegetable oils because it is considered healthier and safe for Paleo diet.

Oil

- Avocado Oil – Avocado oil is oil pressed from an avocado. Many nutritionists claimed that it can help people with high blood cholesterol levels, provides benefits for hair and skin and eventually prevent cancer.

- Butter- Choose with the most natural butter available on the stores because it is made from cows that feed on grass instead of grains that has additional chemicals.

- Coconut oil – Opt for organic coconut oil than the conventional one.

- Olive oil- Considered as one of the best oils, olive oils are beneficial for your every day cooking because it is cheaper and healthier.

Nuts - Nuts are good for snacking in between meals. However, you should stay away from the ones that come in can because it has additional flavourings that may be harmful for your Paleo diet. Opt for raw kinds of nuts that can provide you with energy, sustenance and nourishment.

- Almonds
- Cashews
- Hazelnuts
- Macadamia Nuts
- Pecans
- Pine Nuts
- Pumpkin Seeds
- Sunflower Seeds
- Walnuts

What's Not to Eat on Paleo Diet

Knowing what the foods you should avoid is sometimes easier than identifying the foods that are acceptable on Paleo diet. It is understandable that eating like a cave man can be difficult nowadays because of the wide array of foods available everywhere. Determining the foods you cannot eat can be tricky as well, considering that many products contains chemicals and other preservatives.

With this, the following "Food to Avoid List" may guide you.

- Stay away from Sodas and Sugary Drinks

  Today's sodas contain high amounts of fructose corn syrups and artificial ingredients that have no nutritional value. These are often written as empty carbs, which usually include caffeine that is a not natural substance for humans. For most diet regimen, other than Paleo, drinking soda is also not recommended. This beverage is suspected as primary cause of diabetes and other illness such as high blood pressure, heart disease, obesity and even cancer.

- Avoid foods with Artificial Flavourings

  Artificial ingredients were not around 10,000 years ago. This means that our ancestors never consumed these ingredients. Artificial flavourings were introduced in the last 100 years, some even more recently. If you observe the amount of artificial ingredients found in our foods, you'll be surprised with how much stuff is consumed by most people. Common additives that you should avoid on Paleo include calcium sorbate, nitrates, saccharin, monosodium glutamate, sorbic acide, aspartame, artificial sweeteners, artificial colors and GMO's. Avoiding these foods containing these ingredients may help you obtain a healthier life.

- Partially Hydrogenated Oils are a No-Go

  Early humans did not have the ability or the resources to create oils that can last for months without spoiling. However, many food companies are able to do that, and even developed partially hydrogenated oils. Hydrogenated oils have the ability to stay on your shelf, and extend the shelf life of the foods you will be making with it. Unfortunately, there are claims that partially hydrogenated oils produced trans fat, which is unhealthy for the body.

  As a result, many healthy living advocates argued with food corporations regarding their production of hydrogenated oils that put many Americans at risk. Despite that, companies just developed new ways to hide the trans fat from the Nutritional Information or food labels, or created oils that do not have trans fat but just as bad for the body.

- End your Fast Food Cravings

  There is definitely no Burger King or McDonalds during the Paleolithic Era. Meaning, early humans did not have access to these kinds of foods. In fact, any food that comes out from fast food restaurant may not be acceptable for Paleo. We are not aware of how those foods are engineered, and whether it contains nutrients that might be good for the body. Fast food has a bad reputation following the documentary "Super Size Me" and the book "Fast Food Nation." Fast food usually contains carbohydrates, additives and unnatural ingredients that could be bad for your health.

- Paleo do not Accept Grains

  Grains are not acceptable on Paleo Diet. This is why many dieters considered Paleo diet as Grain-Free Diet or Gluten-Free Diet. Grains are not recommended because during the Paleolithic Era, the diets of our early ancestors were focused on vegetables, fruits and plants, and without a single amount of carbohydrates and grains. Cutting out grains from your diet means you should avoid breads, bagels and other foods containing wheat.

  Many people criticized the Paleo diet because it goes against the Official Food Guide Pyramid endorsed by the US Department of Agriculture. However, many studies revealed that making carbs as primary food source may result in many diseases, such as type 2 diabetes, because eating carbs are associated with insulin resistance and high levels of blood glucose. On the contrary, many have found that avoiding wheat makes them feel better and gives them more energy. People who follow the no-wheat diet can also experience better digestion and loses weight.

- Stop Munching on Junk Foods

A Paleolithic man thrived and survived on natural food sources, which let them live longer without gaining too much weight. However, when Junk Foods were introduced, it became a quick snack that is created to tantalize our taste buds with chemicals from laboratories. Junk food has no nutritional value, and its main purpose is to give us that tantalizing feeling. Kids are not advised to avoid junk food because it is bad for them. It is also because it contains ingredients such as industrial grade salt and ultra sweet sweeteners that may result in child obesity and other negative health effects.

- The Tricky Stuff on Non-Paleo Foods

Dairy, legumes, potatoes and pseudograins are all part of the Standard American Diet. Due to this, it is often hard for Paleo dieters find it's confusing and hard to determine whether each food is acceptable on Paleo or not. You have to be keen on specifying the acceptable and non-acceptable food that belongs to the said categories.

- Dairy

Dairy comes from animals, which make it seem acceptable for Paleo Diet. However, early humans did not have the ability or chance to drink milk, eat yogurt or cheese during their lifetime. Therefore, dairy is actually a non-Paleo food.

Paleo diet supporters also stated that many adult humans are lactose intolerant because their ancestors did not have enough time to adjust with the diet associated with dairy and other cultivated products. More ultimately, paleo diet is all about eating foods produced naturally without added chemicals and artificial flavourings.

- Don't Let Your Body Process Processed Foods

  The number processed foods available in the market are unknown. Usually, foods found in box, and that that says it has longer shelf life, are considered processed. The exceptions only apply to canned food, which is not acceptable on Paleo diet either.

It may be challenging for you to eat on Paleo by means of avoiding processed foods because it accounts for a large majority of food you can find in grocery store or supermarket. Ideally, if you are shopping for food and trying to avoid the processed ones, go to farmer's market for fruits and vegetables then butcher shop for meats.

Chapter 7

Shopping and Creating Meal Plans on Paleo

How to Shop Like a Paleo Expert

For people taking on the Paleo diet, especially beginners, you should be mindful of the food you can and cannot eat. Non-paleo foods include dairy, starches, wheat, legumes and grains. With so many foods not allowed on this diet regimen, you are probably wondering how you are going to enjoy living your life on Paleo. If this diet would be your reason to have a big lifestyle change, the following may teach you how to shop like a Paleo expert.

- Go to the Fresh, Seasonal Produce

You should steer clear of starches such as white potatoes. You cannot snack on fruits as well. Although all fruit and berries are acceptable on the Paleo diet, but choose fruits that are high in sugar such as tangerines, grapes and bananas. These three may help you lose weight more. Pick the green leafy vegetables, which are totally alright on Paleo.

- Enter the Meat Section

It is important for Paleo eaters to consume animal protein and fat from meat. But you should purchase meat that are naturally raised or pasteurized. Experts recommended that animal meat should come from grass-fed and fully pastured animal such as fully pastured pork, grass-fed beef, wild-caught seafood and fully pastured chicken.

- Buy that Healthy Oil for your Cooking

Individuals practicing the Paleo lifestyle are aware of the significance of consuming healthy fats. Healthy fats come from organic and grass-fed animals, which will turn into oils such as olive oil and coconut oil. You can also buy ghee, a clarified butter that was produced by removing its milk solids through boiling.

- Here comes the Flavor

You might think that eating on Paleo diet means eating meals that has little to no flavor. To add some flavor on your homecook Paleo meal, you can use gluten-free Dijon-style mustard, chicken, beef or vegetable broth, coconut milk and other natural dried herb and spices. Almond and coconut flours will be essential for baking and breading, while raw honey and maple syrup will add sweetness to your cooking.

- Fermented Foods are Definitely Okay

The Paleo diet welcomes fermented food because it can do wonders to your digestive system and metabolism. Fermented foods contains natural probiotics that can increase you immunity. Try some kombucha, sauerkraut and kimchi as a side dish.

- Snacking the Paleo way

The diet regiment is all about clean and whole foods that you can prepare at home. Besides this, you should have some convenient snacks with you to contain your cravings just in case. Snacks like dried fruit, raw almonds and cashews, krave jerky and raw almond butter will do.

How to Create your Own Paleo Diet Meal Plans

The Caveman diet is based on the idea of eating like humans did 10,000 years ago during the Paleolithic Era. The benefits of eating on Paleo may include lowering blood sugar levels and sodium intakes. This may sound easy but many people are having a hard time to sustain with the diet regimen. So here's how you can create a solid meal plan without violating the Paleo rules.

Breakfast

If you usually eat eggs for breakfast, you will be glad to know that Paleo diet will allow you have eggs first thing in the morning. Enjoy eggs and bacon that has no additive and low-sodium content. You can eat these together with fresh fruit or veggie smoothie. Include some mixed nuts or nut butter to your smoothie for additional protein. If you love pancakes, you can cook Paleo pancake by using almond milk, coconut flour and mashed banana as ingredients.

Lunch

Because grains and breads are not allowed on Paleo Diet, your beloved sandwich will have to go. Vegetables will play a huge portion during lunch. You can have salad with different vegetables, together with chicken, tuna, scallops, beef, mussels or eggs, in your lunch. Some awesome lunch combination may include a cherry tomato salad and a roasted chicken, a bacon egg and tomato salad, a beef stir fry, or grilled pork chops with spinach.

Dinner

Your diet should not include grains, beans, dairy and processed foods. However, you might still keep your current dinners but with a little changes of healthy ingredients. For example, instead of eating pasta with a Bolognese sauce, you can use spaghetti squash for the sauce. You can use mashed cauliflower as a rice substitute. If you are still uncertain of whether you are following the Paleo diet guidelines, you can have a piece of fish or grilled steak combined with plenty of vegetables.

Snacks

Snacking is important for diet because it can help you sustain your cravings. So instead of munching potato chips in between meals, you can eat nuts, nut betters and celery sticks. Berries, boiled eggs and raw vegetables would be good for your weight loss regimen as well.

You should always remember that portion control is significant on the Paleo Diet. Monitoring your serving sizes and food intake may guarantee that you are eating the right amount of food that is not harmful for your body weight and goals.

One Week Paleo Diet Meal Plan

Consistency is one of the common problem individual's faces when trying to stick with the Paleo diet regimen. There are instances where a person eats a Paleo friendly breakfast and lunch then settled for something unhealthy at the end of the day because they do not know what to make. To solve this problem, here is a 7-day Paleo Diet Meal Plan that you can follow to achieve your goals.

1. Monday
   - Breakfast - Eggs and hash browns made of sweet potato
   - Lunch -Vegetable salad with chopped chicken meat
   - Snack -Paleo Trail Mix (homemade)
   - Dinner -Slowed cook pulled pork (the pork meat should be bought from butchers instead of the grocery store)
2. Tuesday
   - Breakfast – Paleo banana bread (made of coconut or almond flour and bananas)
   - Lunch – Sandwich with bell pepper slices
   - Snack - Avocado
   - Dinner – Taco pie

3. Wednesday
   - Breakfast –Egg with vegetables scramble
   - Lunch –Dinner Leftover (taco pie)
   - Snack- Jerky
   - Dinner –Ground beef stir fry with vegetables
4. Thursday
   - Breakfast –Bacon and eggs, fried in coconut or olive oil
   - Lunch –sandwich in a lettuce leaf with fresh veggies and meats
   - Snack –Cauliflower popcorn
   - Dinner –Grilled fish with spinach
5. Friday
   - Breakfast –Paleo muffins (made of almond flour topped with nuts or sesame seeds)
   - Lunch – Chicken salad with olive oil and nuts
   - Snack –Almond cheese with slices of apple
   - Dinner –Burgers without bun, friend in butter with salsa and vegetables
6. Saturday
   - Breakfast –Steak and eggs
   - Lunch –Cold cut meats and veggies
   - Snack –Roasted pumpkin seeds
   - Dinner –Meat and veggie stir fry
7. Sunday
   - Breakfast –Banana Pancakes
   - Lunch -Soup
   - Snack –Grilled Peaches
   - Dinner –Paleo fried chicken fingers, using coconut oil with kimchi as a side dish

Chapter 8

How to be Successful in your Paleo way of Eating

1. Try to eat like a Caveman for at least 30 days. Paleo diet may show you the positive results within a month if you learn the basics and commit to it.

2. Do the Paleo diet with a friend. Have someone who understands your goals to keep you motivated.

3. Never stop learning. At the beginning, you need to understand different information about Paleo diet. Keep learning and absorb knowledge coming from blogs, news and support groups. Doing so may help you realize how fun it is to have a healthy lifestyle.

4. Get the right tools. You need cooking tools, recipe books and even cooking lessons on Paleo. Go get them to make it easier for your healthy transition.

5. Don't strive for perfection – If you don't get the Paleo 100 percent right, it is okay. Transitioning to the Paleo lifestyle can be difficult at the beginning. Don't be hard on yourself, and just keep going.

6. What other people think of your diet does not matter. You will come across with people saying that Paleo is just too hard. Ignore them and stop the negative vibes from affecting your goal. Prove them wrong.

7. Always have a snack – Nuts, beef jerky and berries would be the foods you can count on when you get hungry between meals. Have a snack to settle your bad food cravings.

8. Think about the long term benefits of Paleo – the benefits of Paleo would be your biggest motivation in sustaining a healthy lifestyle.

9. Fat is not actually bad. – There are diets claiming that fats are bad for your health. It is actually not because there are good fats that can bring numerous benefits to your body.

10. You may adjust to Paleo differently from the others – Your body's reaction during the transition on Paleo would not be the same from other people's body. Despite that, stick with your Paleo plan and achieve your goal.

11. The first week of transition would be the hardest – During those times, find your motivation and hold on to it.

12. Set up your cheat day. Allow yourself to have non-Paleo meal. Although this may mean that you are not following the Paleo diet 100 percent, it is also great to give in with your cravings once in a while, provided that you are 100 percent committed with the diet.

13. Don't deprive yourself of food. When you get hungry, eat. You don't need to count calories on Paleo. Eating natural and whole foods is enough to let your body obtain energy, balanced and health.

14. Learn how to plan and stick to it. Creating a plan would be save you more time. It also ensures that you stay on track. A meal plan may save you from worrying what to eat for breakfast, lunch and dinner.

15. Invest on spices and other Paleo-foods you can store. Some natural spices may be expensive. However, it is a good investment if you want more flavors to your home cook meal.

16. When starting out, keep your cooking simple. You don't have to cook like a chef; you just make meals associated with vegetables, fruits and unprocessed meat. Even if you have zero cooking skills, you will eventually improve by practicing every day.

17. You are not too young or too old for Paleo. If your goal is to have a better health, age would be just a number.

18.   Transition on Paleo gradually. Forcing your body to adjust on Paleo is not advisable. You can ease your way into the transition period instead. Eat 50 percent Paleo on the first week, then the percentage of your Paleo way of eating may increase by 10 percent for the succeeding weeks.

19. Find restaurants that serve Paleo foods. Restaurants that cater for Paleo eaters are best when your friends want to hang out and eat, or when there is something to celebrate.

20.   Physical activity is a must. While Paleo diet allows you to lose weight by eating natural and whole foods, you can add some workout routine or physical activity. Doing so may show better results on your body.

21. Cook extra foods for leftovers. Leftovers make great lunches for the next day.

22.   Ignore what conventional diets are telling you.

23. Take a before and after picture of yourself – Even after eating on Paleo for a month, you will likely see the difference in your body. The results may keep you motivated.

24. Be patient. Helping your body adjust with the new diet may take some time. Just be patient and stay committed with your plan and goals.

25. Cutting off carbs is hard. Yes, giving up carbohydrates would be difficult. However, if doing so allows you to have a perfect physique, health and vibe, why you should not?

Chapter 9

All-time Best Paleo Recipes -- Breakfast, Lunch, Dinner & Desserts

BREAKFAST

Spicy Southwestern Breakfast Bowl

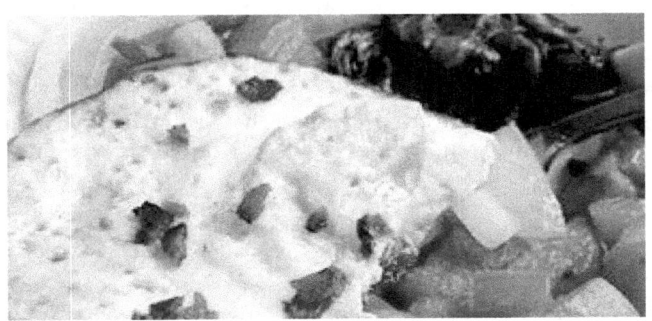

Ingredients

- 2 large sweet potatoes, peeled and diced
- Extra virgin olive oil, for drizzling
- Salt and pepper, to taste
- 1 tsp chili powder
- 2 strips bacon
- 1/2 medium yellow onion, diced
- 1/2 green bell pepper, diced

- 1/2 red bell pepper, diced
- 1 small jalapeno, seeded and diced
- 2-3 cups fresh spinach
- 2 eggs
- 1 tsp ghee
- 1 avocado, pitted and diced, optional

Instructions

- Preheat the oven to 375 degrees F. Place the diced sweet potatoes on a rimmed baking sheet and drizzle with olive oil. Sprinkle with salt, pepper, and chili powder. Bake for 15-20 minutes, turning once.
- Meanwhile, cook the bacon in a skillet over medium heat. Remove to a paper towel-lined plate and crumble. Add the onion, bell peppers, and jalapeno to the skillet and sauté for 5-6 minutes until soft. Lastly add in the spinach and cook until wilted.
- In a separate skillet, melt the ghee. Cook the eggs to desired doneness, seasoning with salt and pepper.
- To assemble, divide the sweet potatoes between two bowls. Top with the veggie mixture, followed by the egg, crumbled bacon, and avocado if using.

Notes

- Servings: 2
- Difficulty: Easy

Paleo Pizza Crust & Breakfast Pizza

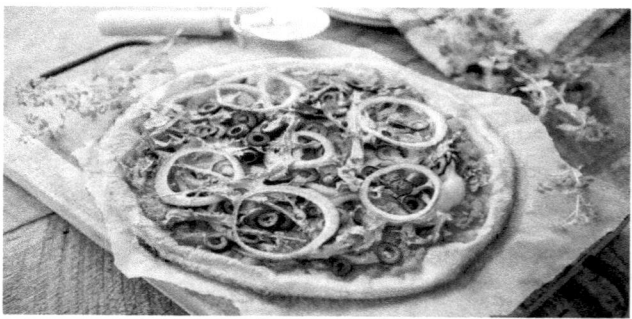

For the crust

- 3 eggs
- 1 cup full-fat canned coconut milk
- 1/2 cup of coconut flour
- 2 tsp of garlic powder
- 1 tsp onion powder

- 1 tsp Italian seasoning
- 1/2 tsp baking soda

For the breakfast pizza

- 3 strips bacon
- 1/4 cup scallions, chopped
- 1-2 tomatoes, sliced thin
- 2 cups spinach
- 4 eggs
- 1 tbsp fresh parsley, chopped

Directions

- Preheat the oven to 375 degrees F. To form the pizza dough, lightly beat the eggs and coconut milk in a bowl. Add in the coconut flour, baking soda, and seasonings and mix into a smooth batter.
- Spread the batter onto a baking sheet lined with parchment paper, using a spatula to smooth into either a circle or rectangle. Bake for 18-20 minutes or until the top is golden brown. Remove from oven. Carefully flip over.
- While the crust is baking, cook the bacon in a skillet over medium heat. Reserving the bacon fat in the pan, set the bacon aside to cool and crumble into pieces. Barely wilt the spinach in the leftover bacon fat.
- Add toppings to the baked crust. Start with bacon, tomato, spinach, and scallions. Carefully crack eggs onto the crust. Sprinkle with parsley. Bake for 12-15 minutes more, just until the egg whites have set. Slice and serve warm.

Notes

- Servings: 4
- Difficulty: Easy

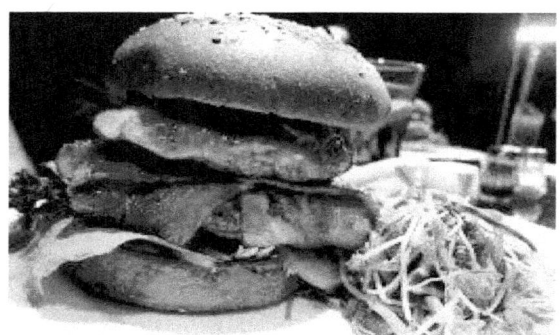

Ingredients

To make the patties, you will need:

- 450g grass fed ground beef
- 1/3 cup crispy lardons *(or 2-3 crispy bacon strips and their drippings)*
- 1 tbsp Dijon mustard
- 3 cloves garlic, chopped
- 1 pastured egg
- ¼ tsp Himalayan or unrefined sea salt
- ¼ tsp freshly cracked black pepper
- ¼ tsp anise seeds
- 1/8 tsp ground clove
- 1 large jalapeño pepper, seeded and very finely chopped
- ¼ cup fresh parsley, finely chopped
- 2 tbsp fresh mint, finely chopped
- 1 tbsp fresh rosemary, finely chopped
- ½ cup sauerkraut, squeezed fairly dry and roughly chopped
- To garnish each burger, you will need:
- 1 fresh kale leaf, torn into several pieces

- 2 slices tomato
- 3 slices avocado
- ¼ cup sauerkraut
- 1 pastured egg, pan fried
- 1 bacon strip, cooked and cut in 2 pieces

INSTRUCTIONS

- Start by cooking the required number of slices of bacon (depending on how many burgers you are making and whether or not you are using cooked bacon in your meat patties) and set aside.
- In a small food processor, add the lardons (or cooked bacon and drippings) Dijon mustard, garlic, egg, salt, pepper, ground clove and anise seeds and process into a paste.
- Add that to a medium mixing bowl along with the ground beef, jalapeño pepper, parsley, mint, rosemary and sauerkraut and knead well with your hands until uniformly blended. Form the meat mixture into 3 or 4 beef patties.
- Preheat your outdoor grill to high.
- Once your grill is nice and hot, lower the heat to medium and place the patties on the grill; cook for about 3-4 minutes per side or until the patties are done to your liking.
- Alternatively, you could also cook the beef patties in a large skillet set over medium-high heat, again, about 3-4 minutes per side.
- While the meat is cooking, pan fry as many eggs as you will require to garnish your burgers.
- To assemble the burgers, start by laying a few pieces of kale at the bottom of a plate. Place the beef patty right over that, followed by the sauerkraut and a few slices of tomatoes and avocado.
- At this point, you might want to insert a toothpick right in the center of the pile to make sure your mile high burger doesn't collapse on you!
- Once everything is good and secure, add the pan fried egg right on top of all that and, finally, place two pieces of cooked bacon right over your egg. BEAUTY!
- Take a nice long look (if you can!) at your beautiful creation and dig in.

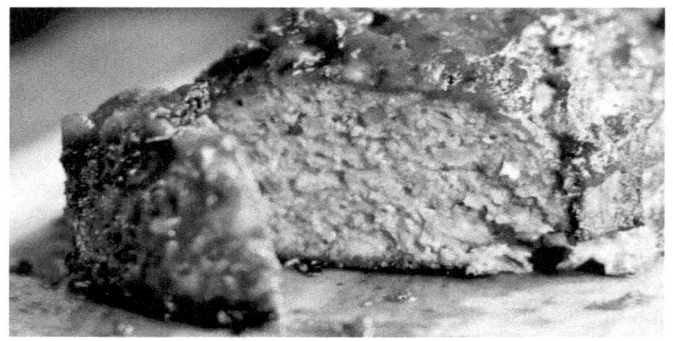

Ingredients
- 2 pounds ground meat – mixture of grass fed beef and/or pork and/or veal
- 10 ounces frozen, chopped spinach
- 1-2 teaspoons oil
- 1 medium onion, finely diced
- 6 ounces mushrooms, finely diced
- 2 carrots, grated or finely diced
- 4 eggs, lightly beaten
- 1/3 cup coconut flour
- 2 teaspoons salt
- 2 teaspoons pepper
- 2 teaspoons onion powder
- 1 teaspoon garlic powder
- 1 teaspoon dried thyme
- 1/4 teaspoon grated nutmeg

Instructions
- Preheat oven to **375 degrees F**

- Thaw the spinach, squeeze out the excess water and set aside.
- Heat a pan on medium heat, add the oil and fry the onions and mushrooms until the onions are translucent and some of the liquid has cooked out of the mushrooms. Set aside to cool.
- Place the ground meat in a large bowl, add the spinach, carrots, mushroom/onion mixture, beaten eggs, coconut flour and all the spices. Use your hands to combine it well but do not overmix.
- Fill 18 regular size muffin tins to the top with the meatloaf mixture. (Greasing the tins may be a good idea if the meat you're using is fairly lean)
- Cook for 20-25 minutes or until internal temperature reaches 160 degrees.
- Allow to cool and use a knife to loosen meatloaves from sides of the pan before removing.
-

Down-Home Brussels Sprout Hash

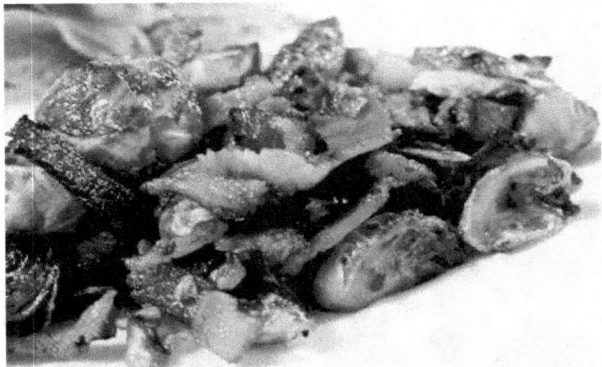

Ingredients

- 3 slices bacon
- 1/2 large butternut squash, peeled, seeded and cubed
- 1/2 small red onion, finely diced
- 1 clove garlic, minced
- 12 oz. Brussels sprouts, stemmed and sliced
- 1 tbsp extra virgin olive oil
- Salt and freshly ground pepper, to taste
- 2-3 eggs, optional

Instructions

- Place the bacon in a pan and cook until crisp. Set aside on a paper towel-lined plate and crumble into pieces. Leave one tablespoon of bacon grease in the pan and dispose of the rest.
- Add the butternut squash, onion, and garlic to the pan and cook for 5-7 minutes, stirring occasionally, until soft. Stir in the Brussels sprouts, along with a tablespoon of olive oil. Season generously with salt and pepper to taste. Sauté for 8-10 minutes until the Brussels sprouts are bright green and fork-tender.
- Add the crumbled bacon back into the pan and stir. Make two or three small wells in the hash and crack an egg into each. Cover and cook until the eggs are set. Serve immediately.

Notes

- Servings: 2-3
- Difficulty: Easy

Paleo Stuffed Breakfast Peppers

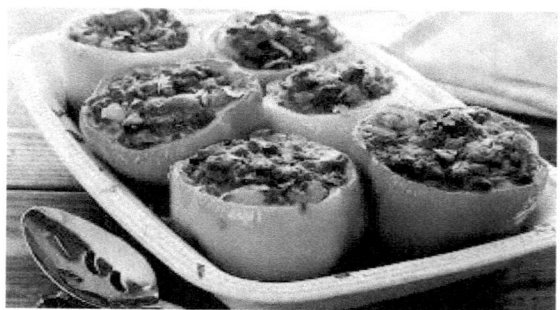

Ingredients

- 2 bell peppers – your choice of color
- 4 eggs
- 1 cup white mushrooms
- 1 cup broccoli
- ¼ tsp cayenne pepper
- Salt and pepper, to taste

Directions

- Preheat oven to 375 degrees Fahrenheit.
- Dice up your vegetables of choice.
- In a medium sized bowl, mix eggs, salt, pepper, cayenne pepper, and vegetables.
- Cut peppers into equal halves. A tip: Try to buy peppers that are symmetrical and have somewhat flat sides – this makes it easier for them to balance while baking.
- Core the peppers so that they're clean enough to add the filling.
- Pour a quarter of the egg / vegetable mix into each pepper halve, adding more vegetables to the top to fill in any empty space.
- Place on baking sheet and cook approximately 35 minutes or until eggs are cooked to your liking.
- Serve and enjoy! I personally like mine with a dash of hot sauce on top.

Notes

This recipe makes 2 servings.

Nutrition Facts Per Serving

- Calories: 186
- Total Fat: 9.4g

- Saturated Fat: 2.8g
- Carbs: 12.1g
- Fiber: 4.0g
- Protein: 14.6g

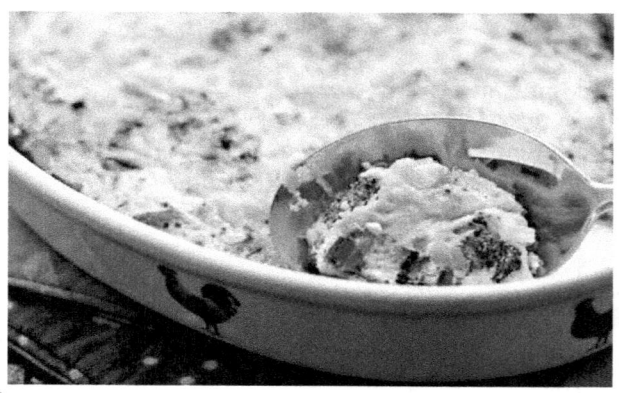

Ingredients

- 3 tbsp of water
- 8 eggs
- 1 tsp of sea salt
- 1 tsp of black pepper
- 2 cups of broccoli chopped small
- 2 cups of red onions
- 2 cups of ham
- 1 tsp of coconut oil

Instructions

- Bake pie dish for 5 minutes on 350 degrees fahrenheit.
- Lightly steam broccoli for a couple of minutes, should turn a pretty bright green. Set aside.
- Saute chopped red onions and chopped ham in coconut oil. If ham is fatty skip coconut oil, the fat will render and be enough.
- Add veggies to lightly baked pie crust.

- Then whisk eggs and water and add over veggies. Water helps make eggs fluffy, so does baking soda. Other recipes I googled use almond and coconut milk. Your pick.
- Bake for 25-30 minutes or until desired firmness.

Notes

Tip: I always undercook food, you can always put it in the oven for longer.

Nutrition Information

Serving size: 4-6

Breakfast Sweet Potato Hash

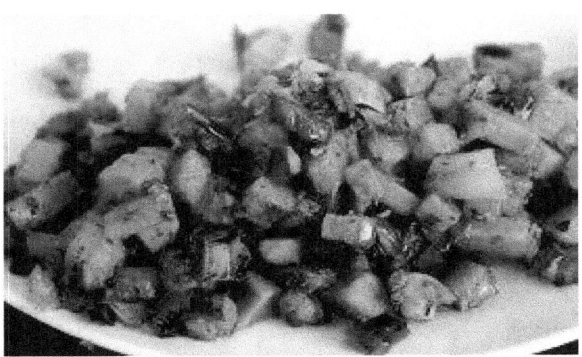

Ingredients

- 1 large onion, sliced
- 3 tbsp olive oil, divided
- 1/2 tbsp ghee
- 2 Italian sausages, diced
- 2 sweet potatoes
- 3 tbsp fresh rosemary
- Salt and freshly ground black pepper, to taste
- 3 eggs

Instructions

- Preheat the oven to 425 degrees F. Line a baking sweet with parchment paper. Heat one tablespoon of olive oil and the ghee in a skillet over medium heat. Add the onions and sprinkle with salt. Cook on low heat for 30-40 minutes, until dark brown and caramelized.
- Meanwhile, peel the sweet potatoes and chop into bite-size pieces. Place into a large bowl with the remaining two tablespoons of olive oil and rosemary.
- In a separate skillet, cook the sausages until browned. Add the cooked onions and sausages to the bowl with the sweet potatoes and toss. Season with salt and pepper.
- Spread out the sweet potato mixture evenly onto the prepared baking sheet. Roast for 30-35 minutes until the potatoes are soft and browned. Either refrigerate overnight at this point or proceed to the next step.
- Place the sweet potato hash into a cast iron skillet and make three small wells to crack the eggs into. Crack eggs into the skillet and season lightly with salt and pepper. Bake for 15-18 minutes at 425 degrees F until the eggs are set.

Notes

- Servings: 4
- Difficulty: Medium

Paleo Breakfast Burritos (Low-Carb)

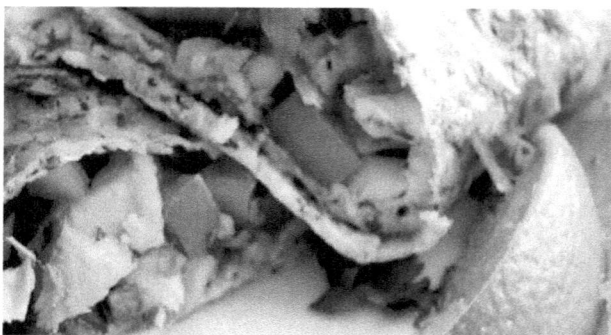

Ingredients

For the tortillas

- 2 eggs
- 2 egg whites
- 1/2 cup water
- 4 tsp ground flaxseed
- Pinch of salt

For the filling

- 1 avocado, diced
- 1/4 cup red bell pepper, finely diced
- 1/4 cup onion, finely diced
- 1/4 cup baked tilapia or other protein
- Handful of spinach leaves
- 1 tsp coconut oil

Instructions

- In a small bowl, whisk together the ingredients for the tortilla. Preheat the oven broiler.
- Heat a 10-inch non-stick skillet over medium heat and coat well with coconut oil spray. Pour half of the tortilla mixture into the pan and swirl to evenly distribute. Using a metal spatula, loosen the edges of the tortilla from the pan. Cook a couple of minutes until golden brown on the bottom, and then carefully slide the spatula under the tortilla to loosen it from the bottom of the pan. Do not flip yet.
- Place the pan under the broiler for 3-4 minutes until the tortilla gets a little bubbly. Remove the tortilla from the pan, setting on a piece of aluminum foil. Repeat with other half of tortilla mixture.
- After the tortillas are done broiling, preheat the oven to 400 degrees F. In a separate small pan, heat the coconut oil over medium heat. Add the onions and peppers and sauté for 5-8 minutes, until soft. Add the spinach into the pan and wilt.
- Place all of the fillings down the center of the tortillas and wrap tightly. Place into the oven for 5-8 minutes to set the shape of the tortilla. Enjoy!

Notes

- Servings: 2
- Difficulty: Medium

Addictive & Healthy Paleo Nachos

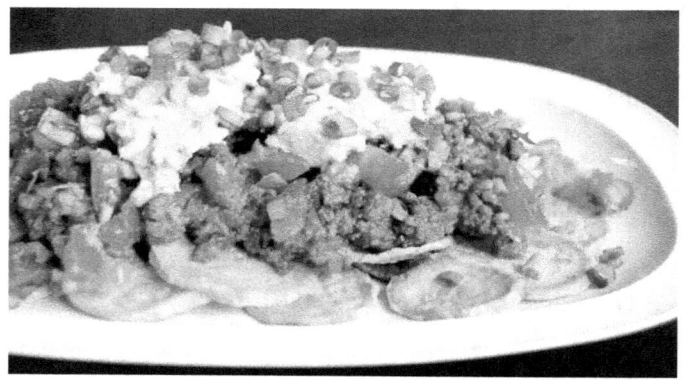

Ingredients

- 2 medium tomatoes, diced and seeded
- 2 tbsp fresh cilantro, chopped
- 1-2 tbsp lime juice
- 2 cups guacamole
- 2 tbsp green onions, chopped

For the sweet potato chips

- 3 large sweet potatoes
- 3 tbsp melted coconut oil
- 1 tsp salt

For the meat

- 1 medium yellow onion, finely diced
- 1 tbsp coconut oil
- 1 green chili, diced
- 1 lb. ground beef
- 2 cloves garlic, minced
- 1 tsp smoked paprika
- 1/2 tsp ground cumin
- 1 tbsp tomato paste
- 12 oz. canned diced tomatoes
- 1 tsp salt
- 1/2 tsp pepper

Instructions

- To make the sweet potato chips, preheat the oven to 375 degrees F. Peel the sweet potatoes and slice thinly, using either a mandolin or sharp knife. In a large bowl, toss them with coconut oil and salt. Place the chips in a single layer on a rimmed baking sheet covered with parchment paper. Bake in the oven for 10 minutes, then flip the chips over and bake for another 10 minutes. For the last ten minutes, watch the chips closely and pull off any chips that start to brown, until all of the chips are cooked.
- While the potato chips are baking, start preparing the beef. Melt the coconut oil in a large skillet over medium heat. Add the onion and chili to the pan and sauté for 3-4 minutes until softened. Add the ground beef and cook for 4-5 minutes, stirring regularly. Add the garlic, diced tomatoes, tomato paste, and remaining spices and stir well to combine. Bring the mixture to a simmer and then turn the heat down to medium-low. Cook, covered, for 20-25 minutes, stirring regularly.
- Stir the chopped tomatoes, lime juice, and cilantro into the beef mixture. Adjust salt and pepper to taste. Remove from heat.
- To assemble the nachos, form a large circle with the sweet potato chips on a platter. Add the beef mixture into the middle of the circle, and then top with guacamole and green onions.

Notes

- Servings: 4-6

- Difficulty: Medium

Paleo Garlic Breadsticks (Just Don't Eat Them All Yourself)

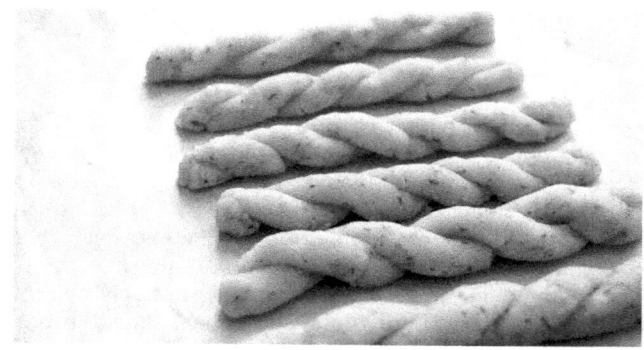

Ingredients

- 1 1/3 cups almond flour
- 1/2 tsp salt
- 2 tbsp coconut oil, melted
- 3 tbsp coconut flour
- 1 clove garlic, minced
- 3 eggs, divided
- 1 tsp dried basil
- 1/2 tsp onion powder
- 1/2 tsp oregano
- 1/2 tsp baking powder
- Ghee, for brushing

Instructions

- Whisk two eggs together in a small bowl and set aside. In a separate bowl, add the almond flour, baking powder, salt, and coconut oil and stir. Add the beaten eggs and stir to combine.
- Add the coconut flour into the bowl, one tablespoon at a time. After each tablespoon let the dough rest for a minute as the flour absorbs. Add the next tablespoon and repeat until you have dough that can be easily kneaded.
- Preheat the oven to 350 degrees F. Line a baking sheet with parchment paper. Roll out the dough onto a separate piece of parchment paper. Working in small handfuls, roll the dough into a long rope. Twist the dough into your shape of choice and place on the baking sheet. Bake for 10 minutes.
- Whisk the remaining egg and add a dash of water. Remove the breadsticks from the oven and brush with the egg wash, and then the minced garlic, basil, onion powder and oregano. Return to the oven and bake for 4-5 minutes more, until golden. Brush with melted ghee before serving.

Notes

- Servings: 4-8 breadsticks, depending on size
- Difficulty: Medium

Eggplant Bolognese with Zucchini Noodles (Low Carb)

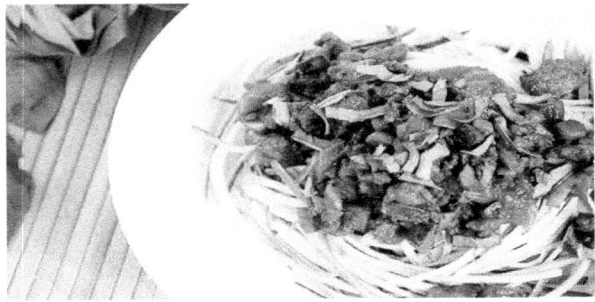

Ingredients

- 1 1/2 lbs. eggplant, diced
- 1/2 lb. ground beef
- 2 tbsp extra virgin olive oil
- Salt and freshly ground pepper
- 1 large yellow onion, chopped
- 3 cloves garlic, minced
- 2 bay leaves
- 4 sprigs thyme
- 1 tbsp tomato paste
- 1/2 cup red wine
- 1 28-oz. can whole peeled plum tomatoes
- 6 leaves fresh basil, chiffonade

Instructions

- Heat the olive oil in a large pan over medium-high heat. Add in the onion and beef and sprinkle with salt and pepper. Cook for 8-10 minutes until the meat is browned. Stir in the eggplant, garlic, bay leaves, and thyme and sauté for an additional 15 minutes.
- Once the eggplant is tender, stir in the tomato paste. Add the wine and scrape any browned bits off the bottom of the pan. Stir in the tomatoes and slightly crush with a spoon. Bring the mixture to a boil, then reduce the heat and simmer for 10 minutes, stirring occasionally. Adjust salt to taste. Serve warm garnished with fresh basil.

Notes

- Servings: 4-6
- Difficulty: Medium

LUNCH

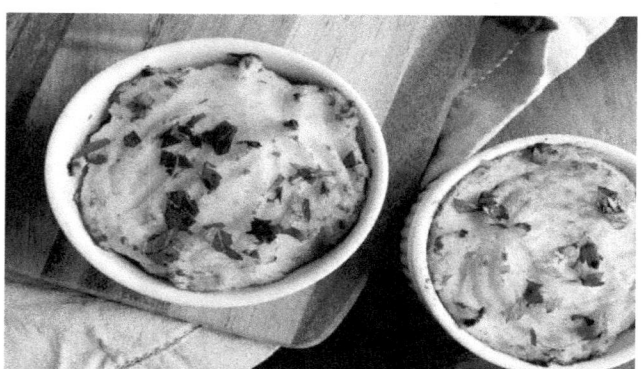

For the top layer

- 1 large head cauliflower, cut into florets
- 2 tbsp ghee, melted
- 1 tsp spicy Paleo mustard
- Salt and freshly ground black pepper, to taste
- Fresh parsley, to garnish

For the bottom layer

- 1 tbsp coconut oil
- 1/2 large onion, diced

- 3 carrots, diced
- 2 celery stalks, diced
- 1 lb. lean ground beef
- 2 tbsp tomato paste
- 1 cup chicken broth
- 1 tsp dry mustard
- 1/4 tsp cinnamon
- 1/8 tsp ground clove
- Salt and freshly ground black pepper, to taste

Instructions

- Place a couple inches of water in a large pot. Once the water is boiling, place steamer insert and then cauliflower florets into the pot and cover. Steam for 12-14 minutes, until tender. Drain and return cauliflower to the pot.
- Add the ghee, mustard, salt, and pepper to the cauliflower. Using an immersion blender or food processor, combine the ingredients until smooth. Set aside.
- Meanwhile, heat the coconut oil in a large skillet over medium heat. Add the onion, celery, and carrots and sauté for 5 minutes. Add in the ground beef and cook until browned.
- Stir the tomato paste, chicken broth, and remaining spices into the meat mixture. Season to taste with salt and pepper. Simmer until most of the liquid has evaporated, about 8 minutes, stirring occasionally.
- Distribute the meat mixture evenly among four ramekins and spread the pureed cauliflower on top. Use a fork to create texture in the cauliflower and drizzle with olive oil. Place under the broiler for 5-7 minutes until the top turns golden. Sprinkle with fresh parsley and serve.

Notes

- Servings: 4
- Difficulty: Medium

Meatball Zucchini Skillet

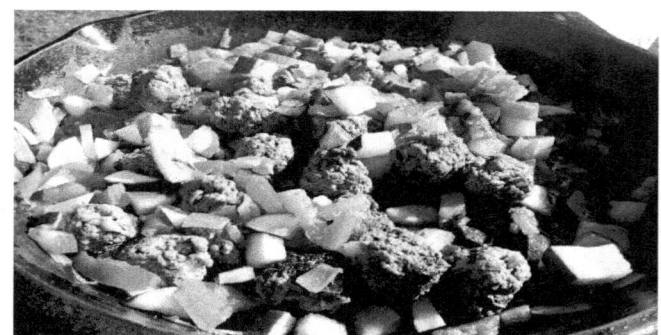

Ingredients:

- Grass-fed butter (coconut oil would also work but the butter gives a great flavor)
- 1/2 large vidalia onion
- 1 pound grass-fed ground beef (if using lean beef you may need to add an egg to hold the meatballs together)
- 1 1/2 tsp garlic powder
- 1 1/2 tsp onion powder
- 1 tsp Italian seasoning
- 2 medium zucchinis
- 2 medium tomatoes
- sea salt and pepper to taste

Directions:

- Put your skillet on medium-high heat.
- Then dice your onions and add them to the skillet with 1-2 tbsp of butter. Saute for around 5 minutes until translucent.
- While the onions are cooking take your grass-fed ground beef and roll them into small 1 1/2 inch balls (we came up with about 20). Add the meatballs to the pan and cook for around 10 minutes, stirring them occasionally, flipping them over to get even cooking, and adding any additional butter if needed to prevent sticking (<< we didn't need any since our beef had a higher fat content, but if you are using lean ground beef the extra butter may be necessary).

- When the beef is cooking wash and dice up the zucchini and tomatoes. Add those to the skillet next along with the seasonings.
- Place a lid over the skillet and reduce to medium heat. Cook for around 5 minutes then remove the lid, stir and put it back on top of the skillet. We cooked the beef and vegetables for another 5 minutes or so until tender, but keep checking them to see when they are done for you.
- Finally plate up some of the meatballs and vegetables topping with salt and pepper as desired.

Paleo Pulled Pork Sliders

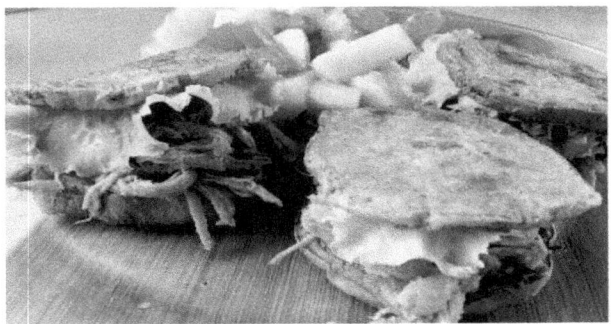

Ingredients

- Large pork roast
  1 large onion, sliced
  3 minced garlic cloves
  2 tsp cumin
  2 tsp chili powder
  1 tsp pepper
  2 tsp oregano
  1 tsp paprika

1/2 tsp cayenne pepper
1/2 tsp cinnamon
- 2 tsp sea salt
juice of 1 lime
juice of 1 lemon

Instructions

- Stir together the spices and rub all over the roast. Lay the onion slices down on the bottom of the slow cooker, and squeeze half of the fruit juices in. Put the roast in the crockpot and squeeze the remaining lime and lemon juice over it. Cook on low overnight or throughout the day about 8 hours (you really can't overcook it to be honest). When done, shred it with two forks until it's completely 'pulled'.

The "Buns"

1 large sweet potato (try to go for a nice evenly round one, remember the diameter will be the size of your sliders)
2 tbsp coconut oil
3. 1/4 tsp cumin
4. 1/4 tsp paprika
5. dash of sea salt

Instructions

- Slice the sweet potato into 1/4″ thick rounds. Lay them out on a parchment paper-lined cookie sheet.

- Brush each slice with coconut oil and sprinkle with the spices, then flip and do the same on the other side.

- Bake at 425 degrees Farenheit for 35 minutes until golden brown on the outside and cooked all the way through, flipping halfway through. You may need to crank it up to 450 if your oven isn't nice and sizzly.

- Top a patty with pulled pork, and add any other toppings or sauces you'd like (I just used some lettuce from our garden).

- Finish with the top patty and enjoy your delightful little sliders! ☺

Crock-Pot Roast

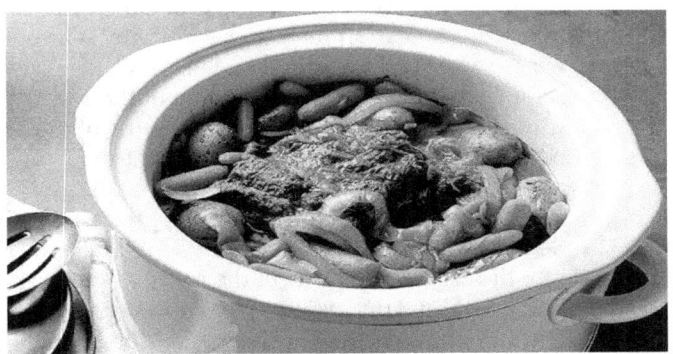

Ingredients

- 4 lb (1816g) beef chuck roast
- 1 tbsp (14g) light oil (for sautéing ... such as coconut, olive or ghee)
- 1 cup (232g) red wine, good quality
- 4 each (12g) garlic cloves
- 10 sprigs (10g) fresh thyme
- 1 each (.64g) bay leaf
- 1 large (72g) carrot, peeled and cut into chunks
- 2 each (101g) celery ribs, cut into chunks
- 1 small (110g) onion, cut into chunks
- 1 small (420g) head cauliflower, leaves removed and cut into florets
- salt and fresh cracked pepper, to taste

Instructions:

- Turn on your slow cooker, setting it to low.
- Season your beef with a good layer and salt and pepper.
- Heat a large sauté pan or skillet over medium high heat. Add your oil to the pan and swirl it around. Quickly add your beef to the pan and sear it, until a nice brown crust has formed. Flip it over and sear the other side. Continue flipping it, until all sides have been properly seared. Add your beef to the crock pot.
- Pour your red wine into the still very hot pan, with all the "stuff" stuck to the bottom. This should QUICKLY boil, releasing some of those little flavor morsels into the hot wine. Swirl the pan around and use a wooden spoon to scrape anything else off the bottom of the pan, into the wine. Pour the wine mixture over the top of the beef.
- Add your garlic, thyme and bay leaves to the slow cooker, making sure it's pushed into the liquid.
- Add the rest of the vegetables, except the cauliflower. Season with a bit of salt and pepper. Again, push these into the areas on the side of the roast, as much as possible. You don't want much of it covering the roast. You want most of the veggies on the sides, surrounding the roast. As this all cooks, the meat and veggies will shrink, releasing their juices, creating an AMAZING flavor, as well as creating its own natural juices, in which to cook! Getting everything as close to the bottom of the pot, as is possible, will help this process along.
- 7. Add the lid and allow the ingredients to cook for 8 hours.
- 8. After 8 hours, add your cauliflower to the pot and push the florets under the surface of the liquid, as much as possible. Season with a bit of salt and pepper. Cover and allow to cook for 20 minutes.
- 9. Serve!

Tuna Avocado Lettuce Wraps (Makes the Perfect Lunch)

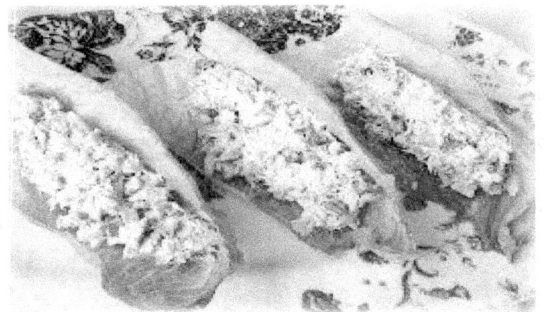

Ingredients

- 1 can tuna
- ½ very ripe avocado
- 2 tbsp paleo mayo
- ¼ cup green olives
- 2 tbsp diced green chiles
- 1 scallion
- 2 large leaves of green leaf lettuce (or your favorite green!)
- This recipe serves two, but is so good you just may eat the whole thing yourself.

Instructions

- Cut olives in half and dice scallion.
- Mash the avocado until it's a creamy consistency, and then mix with paleo mayonnaise.
- Add in the tuna, olives, scallion, and diced green chiles to the avocado-mayonnaise mixture.
- Place one scoop of tuna salad into a large leaf of lettuce, wrap, and enjoy!

Finger Lickin' Chipotle Meatballs

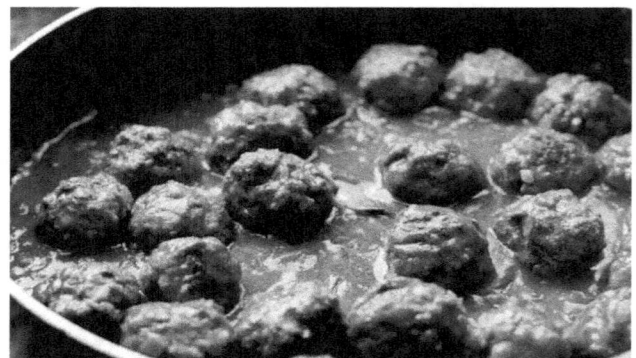

Ingredients

- 1 large, deep frying pan
- 1 large brown onion, peeled and diced finely
- 1 tsp of lard or ghee (clarified butter)

For the meatballs mix

- 800g of grass fed beef mince (1.8 pounds ground beef)
- 3 medium dried chipotle chilies (tinned chipotle can also be used), seeds out
- 2 tbsp chopped fresh coriander (cilantro)
- 2 large garlic cloves, finely diced
- 1 tsp ground coriander seed or powder
- 1 tsp ground cumin seed or powder
- 1 tsp sweet or medium paprika
- 1 tbsp virgin olive oil
- 1 ½ tsp of sea salt
- 2 tbsp lard (I used a mix of lard and ghee)

- ½ of the onion mentioned above
- 2 garlic cloves, finely chopped

- 2 medium chipotle chilies, seeds out
- ½ tsp ground coriander seed or powder
- 1 tsp ground cumin seed or powder
- ½ tsp paprika
- 2 bay leaves
- 400g of diced tomatoes or tomato puree (about 1 ½ cups)
- ½ tsp sea salt

Instructions

- If using dried chipotle chilies, place in hot water for at least an hour before using to rehydrate.
- Sauté the onion in lard or ghee for 3-5 minutes, until translucent. Use half of the onion in the meatball mix and reserve the rest for the sauce.
- While onion is cooking, pre-chop other ingredients for the meatballs. Slice the chipotle chilies in half and remove the seeds. Chop or grind with mortar and pestle.
- Combine beef mince with half of the cooked onion, chopped garlic, chipotle chilies, paprika, cumin, coriander seed, salt and olive oil. Combine and knead with your hands. Using clean, wet hands roll the mix into small balls (somewhere between a walnut and a golf ball size). Set aside until ready to cook.
- Preheat a dollop of lard in the large frying pan until sizzling hot. Cook the meatballs on medium/high heat for 3 minutes on each side, until well browned.
- Add the rest of the cooked onion, garlic, two chopped chilies and sauce spices to the pan with the meatballs. Stir through and add the tomato puree. Combine and cook for 8-10 minutes uncovered, stirring frequently to make sure the meatballs cook evenly and the sauce is well combined. Taste for salt. Drizzle with a little lime juice before serving.

Preparation time: 20 minutes

Cooking time: 20 minutes

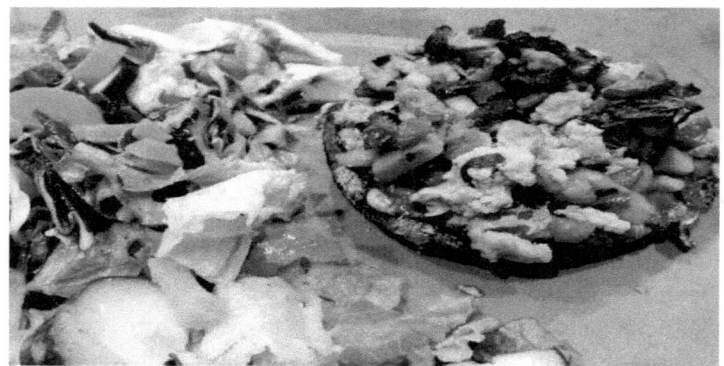

Ingredients

For the Filling:

slices bacon, chopped into 4 or 5 large pieces
½ fennel bulb, roughly chopped
1/2 cup brussels sprouts, bottoms trimmed off and halved
4. 2 garlic cloves
1 tsp each of dried rosemary, sage and oregano

Additional Ingredients:
2, ½ lb sirloin steaks
Salt and pepper, to taste
2 cups Brussels sprouts (about ¾ lb), bottoms trimmed off and quartered
½ fennel bulb, cut into thick slices
1 tsp olive oil
2 or 3 fennel fronds

Directions

Preheat oven to 375F.
Add all filling ingredients to a food processor. Process until it forms a thick

paste.

Pound out steaks using a mallet until they are about ½ inch thick.

Spread half of the filling on each steak. Roll steaks up, using a few toothpicks to secure.

Place sirloin rolls in a large roasting pan and sprinkle with salt and pepper.

Toss Brussels sprouts and fennel slices in a large bowl with olive oil, salt and pepper.

Spread brussels sprouts and fennel slices around sirloin rolls in the roasting pan.

Roast for 35-40 minutes, until steak is cooked to desired level and vegetables begin to brown. If steak is done and veggies need to cook a bit longer, remove the steak from the pan and let it rest while you cook the veggies for an additional five minutes or so.

Let steak rest for 5 minutes before slicing. Garnish with fennel fronds.

Easy Paleo Spaghetti Squash & Meatballs

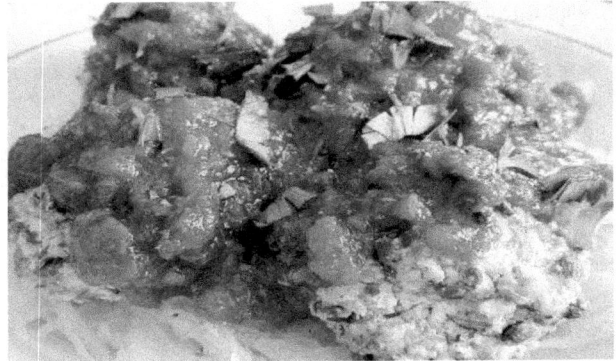

Ingredients

- One medium spaghetti squash.
- One pound of ground Italian sausage.
- One can of tomato sauce, I used a 14 ounce can.
- 2 tbsp of hot pepper relish (optional).
- 4 to 6 cloves of garlic, whole.
- 2 tbsp of olive oil.
- Italian seasoning (Oregano, Basil, Thyme) to taste, I used about 2 tsp

Instruction

- Make sure you use a large 6 quart slow cooker for this recipe.
- Dump your tomato sauce, olive oil, garlic, hot pepper relish and Italian seasoning into your slow cooker and stir well.
- Cut your squash in half and scoop out the seeds.
- Place your 2 squash halves face down into your slow cooker.
- Roll your ground sausage into meatballs, then fit as many as you can in the sauce around the squash. I was able to work in about a half pound worth.

- Cook on High for 3 hours or cook on low for 5 hours.
- Use a large fork to pull the "spaghetti" out of your squash, then top with your meatballs and sauce.
- Garnish with parsley if you feel fancy, and enjoy!

Paleo Crock Pot Cashew Chicken

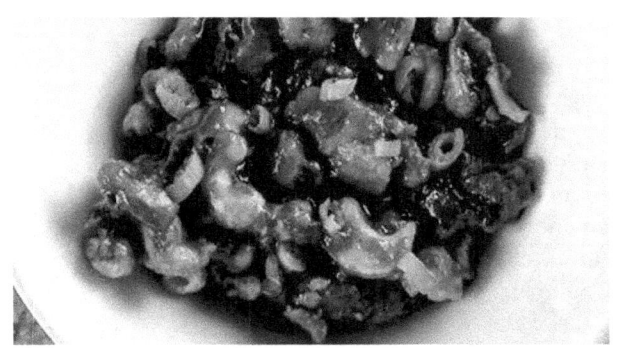

Ingredients

- 1/4 cup arrowroot starch
- 1/2 tsp. black pepper
- 2 lbs. chicken thighs, cut into bite-size pieces
- 1 tbs. coconut oil
- 3 tbs. coconut aminos
- 2 tbs. rice wine vinegar
- 2 tbs. organic ketchup (tomato paste would work also)
- 1/2-1 tbs. palm sugar
- 2 minced garlic cloves
- 1/2 tsp. minced fresh ginger
- 1/4-1/2 red pepper flakes
- 1/2 cup raw cashews

Instructions

1. Place starch and black pepper in a large Ziploc bag. Add chicken pieces and seal; toss to thoroughly coat meat.
2. Melt coconut oil in a large skillet or wok. Add chicken and cook for about 5 minutes until brown on all sides. Remove and add to crock pot.
3. Mix coconut aminos through red pepper flakes in a small bowl. Pour mixture over chicken and toss to coat. Put lid on crock pot and cook on low for 3-4 hours.
4. Stir cashews into chicken and sauce before serving.

Spicy
Cooker
Chili

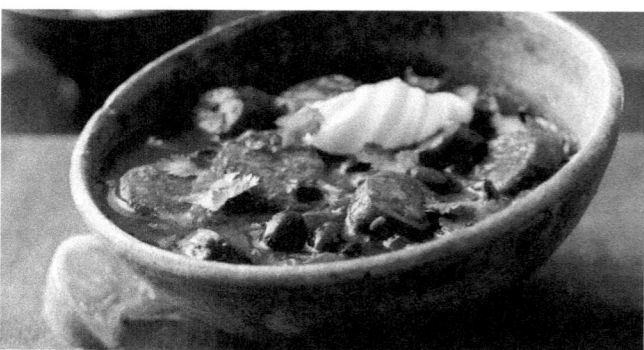

Slow
Chorizo

Ingredients

- 1 pound of grass fed beef
- 2 fresh chorizo sausages, casings removed (about 1/2 pound)
- 1 onion, diced
- 1 teaspoon of minced garlic
- 1 15 oz can of tomato sauce
- 1 15 oz can of diced tomatoes
- 1 can of rotel, I used hot

- 2 chipotle peppers in adobo, chopped
- 2 Tablespoons of chili powder
- 1 Tablespoon of cumin
- salt and pepper to taste

Instructions

- brown off all the meat in a skillet
- drain and toss in the crock pot
- in the same skillet add onions and garlic and cook just long enough to get some color on those onions (you may skip this step and just toss it in the crock pot, but I just personally like to get some color on the onions before adding them in)
- toss remaining ingredients in the crock pot and stir together

- cook on low for 6-8 hours or on high for 4-6 hours
- top with diced avocado, minced red onion and cilantro to serve

Perfect Tomatillo Salsa Verde

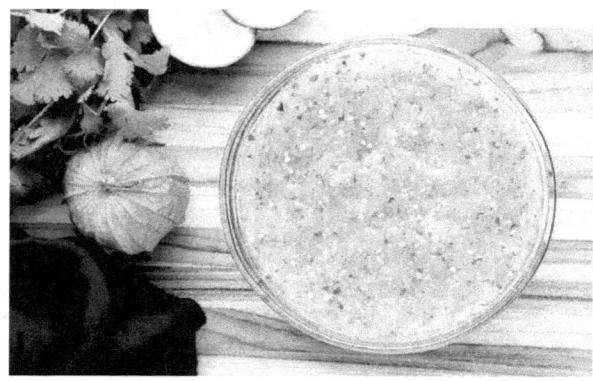

Ingredients

- 1 lb. tomatillos, husked
- 1/2 medium onion, coarsely chopped

- 1 clove garlic, minced
- 1 Serrano pepper, seeded and coarsely chopped
- 1/4 cup fresh cilantro, chopped
- Juice of 1/2 lime
- 1 tsp salt

Instructions

- Place the tomatillos in a saucepan and cover with water. Broil to a boil, then turn the heat to simmer for 5 minutes. Remove with a slotted spoon.
- Place the tomatillos and the remaining ingredients into a food processor and puree until smooth. Adjust salt to taste. Add water if

necessary to reach desired consistency. Place in the refrigerator to chill before serving.

Notes

- Servings: about 2 cups
- Difficulty: Easy

Homemade Herbed Paleo Mayonnaise

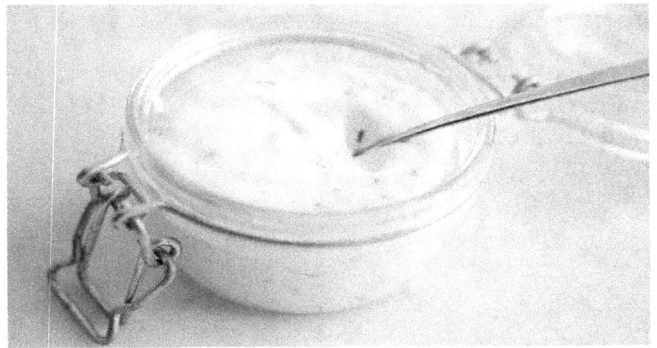

Ingredients

- 1 egg (at room temperature)
- 2 tbsp lemon juice
- 1 tsp rosemary
- 1 tsp oregano
- ½ tsp sea salt
- 1 cup light olive oil (not EVOO – the flavor will be too strong)
- This recipe will make approximately 24 1tbsp servings

Directions

- Add egg, lemon juice, rosemary, oregano, and sea salt to a mixing bowl.
- Whisk together with an electric mixer on low until well blended. Don't turn off the mixer at any point during this process.
- While still whisking, slowly add in your olive oil. Slow is the key word here. Like, one little drizzle at a time slow. Slowly but surely, you'll see the emulsion start to form. Once you see the emulsion forming, continue to add in your olive oil just as slowly until your mayonnaise reaches the desired consistency.
- Refrigerate in a glass jar and enjoy! Will last in the fridge approximately one week.

Nutrition Facts Per Serving

- Calories: 56
- Total Fat: 6.5g
- Saturated Fat: 1.0g
- Carbs: 0.1g
- Protein: 0.2g

Homemade Paleo Ketchup with a Kick

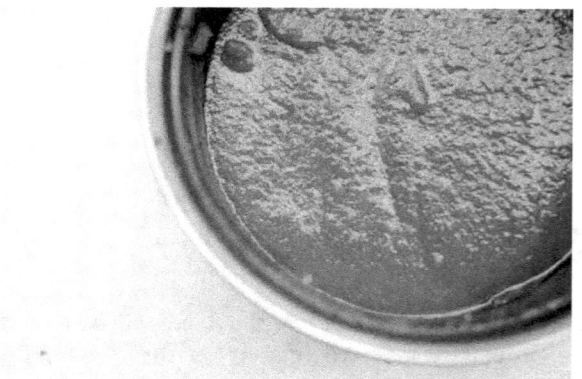

Ingredients

- 1 12 oz can tomato paste
- 1 cup water
- 2 tbsp vinegar
- ½ tsp salt
- ½ tsp curry powder
- ½ tsp garlic powder
- This recipe makes approximately 32 oz of ketchup, or 64 1tbsp servings.

Directions

- Mix all ingredients in a sauce pan and bring to boil on medium-high heat.
- Reduce heat to medium-low and simmer while stirring frequently until flavors have blended. (Add more water for thinner ketchup, add less water for thicker)
- Transfer to a glass jar and cool before serving.

Nutrition Facts Per Serving

- Calories: 5
- Total Fat: 0.0g
- Sodium: 21mg
- Carbs: 1.0g
- Protein: 0.7g

Homemade Paleo Honey Mustard from Scratch

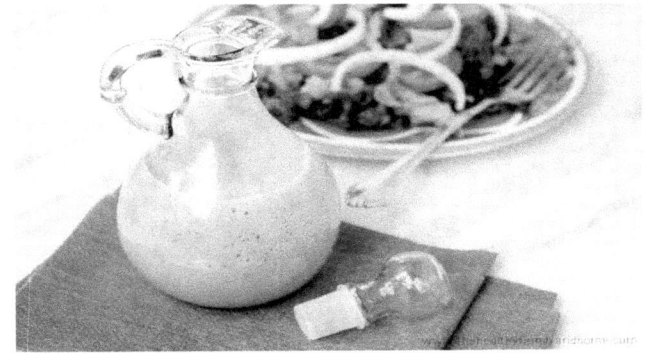

Ingredients

- 1/4 cup mustard powder
- 1/4 cup water
- 3 tbsp honey
- Sea salt, to taste

Instructions

- Place the mustard powder and water in a bowl and stir until combined. Add salt and honey to taste. Let stand for at least 15 minutes before serving.

Notes

- Servings: about 1/2 cup
- Difficulty: Easy

Melt In Your Mouth Slow Cooker Beef Brisket

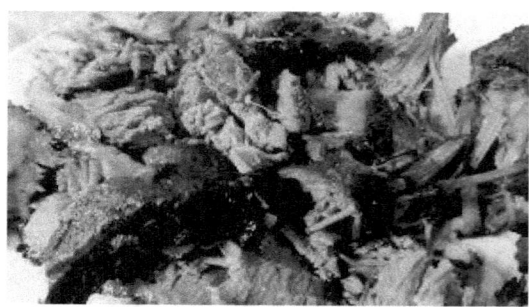

Ingredients

- 2 lbs. beef brisket
- 1 large onion, chopped
- 6 carrots, diced
- 8 oz. mushrooms, sliced
- 6 cloves garlic, peeled and sliced
- 3 cups beef broth
- 4 fresh thyme sprigs
- 1/2 tsp salt
- Freshly ground pepper

Instructions

- Add the onion, carrots, mushrooms, and garlic to the slow cooker. Pour in the beef broth and then add the brisket. Sprinkle with salt and pepper and add the thyme. Cover and cook on low heat for 8-16 hours, until the meat is tender.

Notes

1. Servings: 4
2. Difficulty: Easy

Bacon-Wrapped Roasted Asparagus

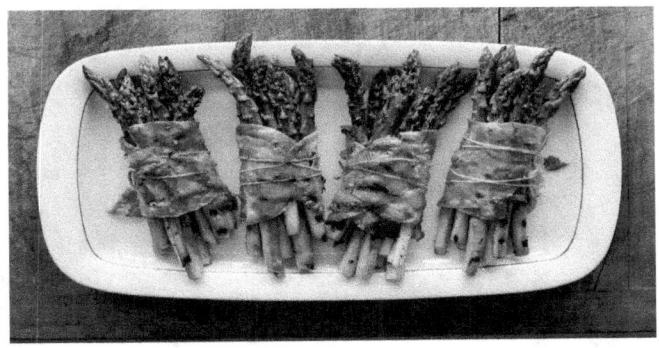

Ingredients

- 1 bunch asparagus, ends trimmed
- 4 pieces bacon
- Extra virgin olive oil
- Salt and pepper, to taste
- Maple syrup, optional

Instructions

- Preheat the oven to 400 degrees F. Place the bacon in a large skillet. Cook for about 3 minutes per side, until the bacon gets just a little crisp. Remove to a paper towel-lined plate.
- Line a rimmed baking sheet with aluminum foil or a Silpat. Wash and dry the asparagus and then place it on the baking sheet. Drizzle with olive oil and toss to coat. Sprinkle with salt and pepper.
- Divide the asparagus into 4 small bundles. Wrap a piece of bacon around each bundle of asparagus and place on the baking sheet. Brush the bacon with maple syrup if desired. Bake for 10-12 minutes, or until the bacon is crisp. Serve immediately.

Notes

- Servings: 4
- Difficulty: Easy

Simple Piccata 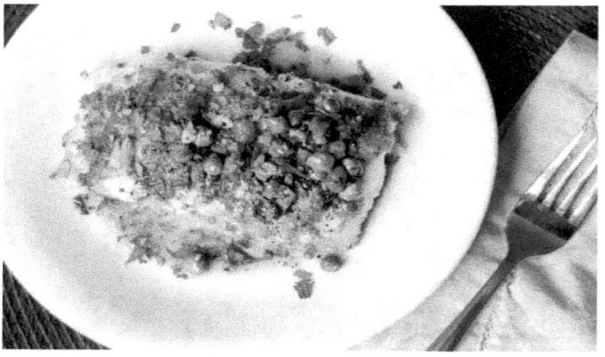 Cod

Ingredients

- 1 lb. cod fillets
- 1/3 cup almond flour
- 1/2 tsp salt
- 2-3 tbsp extra virgin olive oil
- 2 tbsp grapeseed oil, divided
- 3/4 cup chicken stock
- 3 tbsp lemon juice
- 1/4 cup capers, drained
- 2 tbsp fresh parsley, chopped

Instructions

- Stir the almond flour and salt together in a shallow bowl. Rinse off the fish and pat dry with a paper towel. Dredge the fish in the almond flour mixture to coat.
- Heat enough olive oil to coat the bottom of a large skillet over medium-high heat along with one tablespoon grapeseed oil. Working in batches, add the cod and cook for 2-3 minutes per side to brown. Remove to a plate and set aside.
- Add the chicken stock, lemon juice, and capers to the same skillet and scrape any browned bits off the bottom. Simmer to reduce the sauce by almost half. Remove from heat and stir in the remaining tablespoon of grapeseed oil.
- To serve, divide the cod onto plates, drizzle with the sauce, and sprinkle with parsley.

Notes

- Servings: 2-3
- Difficulty: Medium

Paleo BLT Frittata

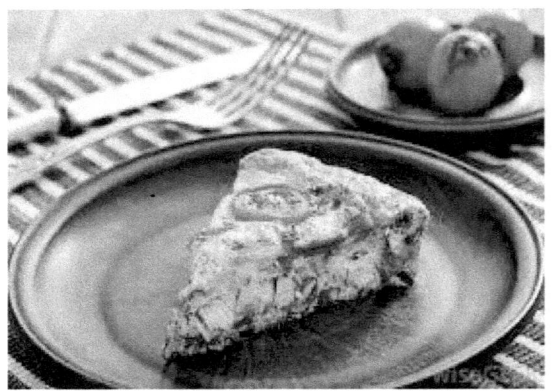

Ingredients

- 8 eggs
- 4 slices bacon, cooked and chopped
- 3-4 cups spinach (or other greens of your choice)
- 1 large tomato, sliced and seeded
- 1 tbsp almond milk
- 1/2 tsp salt
- 1/4 tsp pepper
- 2 tbsp chopped fresh basil
- 1 tbsp extra virgin olive oil

Instructions

- Preheat oven to 400 degrees F. In a medium bowl, whisk together the eggs, milk, basil, salt and pepper. Set aside.
- Heat olive oil in a 10-inch nonstick skillet over medium heat. Add greens and cook 3-4 minutes until wilted. Add in bacon and stir.
- Add egg mixture to the pan and place tomatoes on top. Using a spatula, occasionally lift the edges to allow uncooked egg to run under. When the frittata has set, transfer to the oven and cook for 12-

15 minutes or until egg is cooked through. Cut into wedges and serve warm.

Notes

- Servings: 5
- Difficulty: Easy

Spaghetti Squash Shrimp Scampi (Grain-Free & Low Carb)

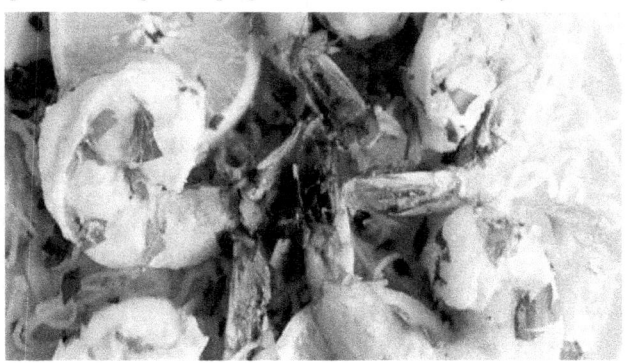

For the "pasta"

- 1 spaghetti squash
- Extra virgin olive oil, for drizzling
- Salt and pepper
- 1 tsp dried oregano
- 1 tsp dried basil

For the shrimp scampi

- 8 oz. shrimp, peeled and deveined
- 3 tbsp butter
- 1 tbsp extra virgin olive oil
- 2 cloves garlic, minced
- Pinch of red pepper flakes

- Salt and pepper, to taste
- 1 tbsp fresh parsley, chopped
- Juice of 1 lemon
- Zest of half a lemon

Directions

- Preheat the oven to 400 degrees F. Place squash in the microwave for 3-4 minutes to soften. Using a sharp knife, cut the squash in half lengthwise. Scoop out the seeds and discard. Place the halves, with the cut side up, on a rimmed baking sheet. Drizzle with olive oil and sprinkle with seasonings. Roast in the oven for 45-50 minutes, until you can poke the squash easily with a fork. Let it cool until you can handle it safely. Then scrape the insides with a fork to shred the squash into strands.
- After removing spaghetti squash from the oven, melt the butter and olive oil in a skillet over medium heat. Add in the garlic and sauté for 2-3 minutes. Then add in the shrimp, salt, pepper, and a pinch of red pepper flakes. Cook for 5 minutes, until the shrimp is cooked through. Remove from heat and add in desired amount of cooked spaghetti squash. Toss with lemon juice and zest. Top with parsley to serve.

Honey Balsamic Roasted Brussels Sprouts

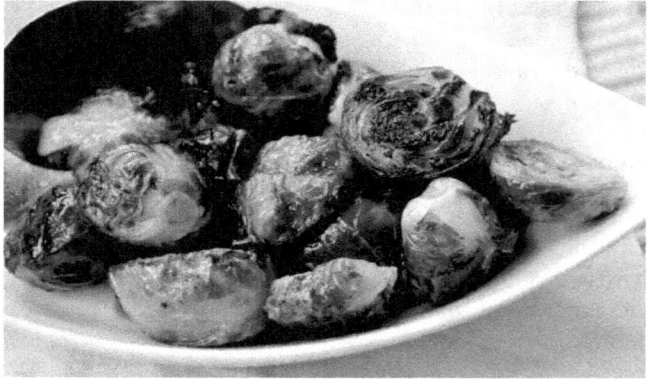

Ingredients

- ½ lb Brussels sprouts
- 1 tbsp olive oil
- 3 tbsp balsamic vinegar
- 1 tbsp honey
- 1 tsp garlic powder
- 1 tsp cayenne pepper
- sea salt & black pepper, to taste
- This recipe makes 2 servings

Directions

- Preheat oven to 450 degrees Fahrenheit. Line a baking sheet with foil and spray with non-stick cooking spray or spread with a light layer of olive oil.
- Halve the Brussels sprouts. Place in a mixing bowl and add in the olive oil, balsamic vinegar, honey, and spices. Toss with hands until fully coated.
- Pour Brussels sprouts onto baking sheet in one layer.
- Bake for 20 minutes, or until golden brown.
- Serve and enjoy! I like to sprinkle another bit of sea salt on them before eating.

Nutrition Facts per serving

- Calories: 153
- Fat: 7.5g
- Saturated Fat: 1.1g
- Carbs: 20.5g
- Fiber: 4.7g
- Protein: 4.2g

Paleo Shrimp Fried "Rice"

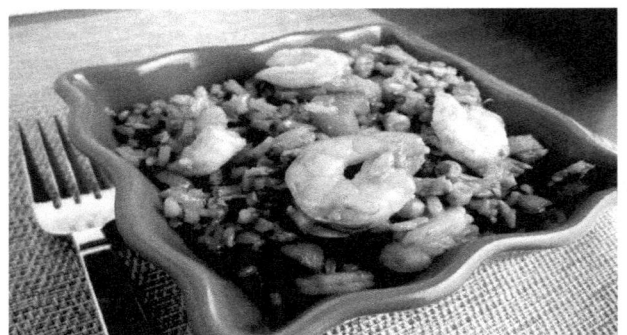

Ingredients

- 1 tbsp coconut oil
- 1 cup white onion, finely chopped
- 2 cloves garlic, minced
- 8 oz. shrimp, peeled and deveined
- 1 medium carrot, chopped
- 1/2 cup peas
- 1/4 cup red bell pepper, finely chopped
- 2 cups cooked cauliflower rice
- 2 eggs, beaten
- Salt and pepper, to taste

Instructions

- Heat a wok or large pan over medium-high heat. Melt the coconut oil and add the onion and garlic to the pan. Cook for 3-4 minutes until the onion starts to soften. Add the shrimp and cook for 1 minute.
- Add the carrot, peas, and bell pepper to the pan. Cook for 3-4 minutes, and then stir in the cauliflower rice. Clear a circle in the center of the pan and pour in the beaten eggs. Stir to scramble the eggs and then combine with the other ingredients. Season with salt and pepper to taste.

Notes

- Servings: 2

- Difficulty: Easy

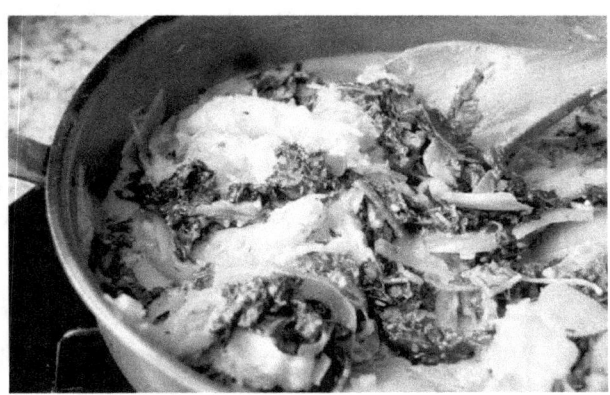

Ingredients

- 1 lb. Italian sausage
- 1 medium spaghetti squash, halved and seeded
- Extra virgin olive oil, for drizzling
- 1 large bunch of kale, de-stemmed, and chopped
- 1/2 red onion, sliced thin
- 1/3 cup chicken broth
- 1/2 cup coconut milk
- 1 clove garlic, minced
- 2 tsp Italian seasoning
- Salt and freshly ground pepper, to taste

Instructions

- Preheat the oven to 400 degrees F. Place the squash in the microwave for 3-4 minutes to soften. Using a sharp knife, cut the squash in half lengthwise. Scoop out the seeds and discard. Place the halves, with the cut side up, on a rimmed baking sheet. Drizzle with olive oil and sprinkle with salt and pepper. Roast in the oven for 45-50 minutes, until you can poke the squash easily with a fork. Let it cool until you can handle it safely. Then scrape the insides with a fork to shred the squash into strands.

- Meanwhile, melt the coconut oil in a large oven-safe skillet over medium heat. Add the sausage and brown. Once cooked through, remove to a plate. In the same skillet, add the onion and sauté for 3-4 minutes. Next add the garlic, Italian seasoning, and kale and cook for 2-3 minutes to slightly wilt the kale. Pour in the chicken broth and coconut milk and simmer for an additional 2-3 minutes. Remove from heat.
- Stir in the cooked sausage. Add the spaghetti squash into the skillet and stir well to combine. Bake for 15-18 minutes, until the top has slightly browned. Serve hot.

Notes

- Servings: 4
- Difficulty: Medium

Basic Balsamic Steak Marinade

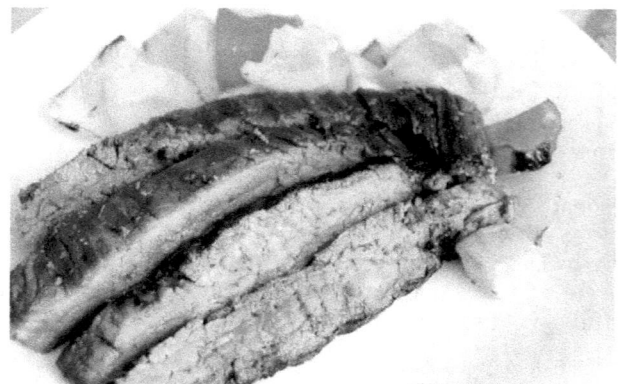

Ingredients

- 1 lb. flank steak
- Salt and pepper
- 2 cloves garlic, minced
- 1/2 tbsp oregano
- 1/2 tbsp rosemary
- 1 tsp Paleo mustard
- 1/4 cup balsamic vinegar
- 1 tsp honey
- 1/2 cup extra virgin olive oil

Instructions

- Stir together the garlic, oregano, rosemary, mustard, vinegar, honey, and olive oil.
- Salt and pepper the steak and place in a shallow dish, then pour the marinade over the steak. Cover and place in the refrigerator for 3-12 hours.
- To cook the steak, heat the grill to medium and cook each side approximately 4-5 minutes, or until desired doneness. Let stand for about 5 minutes before slicing and serving.

Notes

- Servings: 3
- Difficulty: Medium

Rosemary Beets with Garlicky Kale

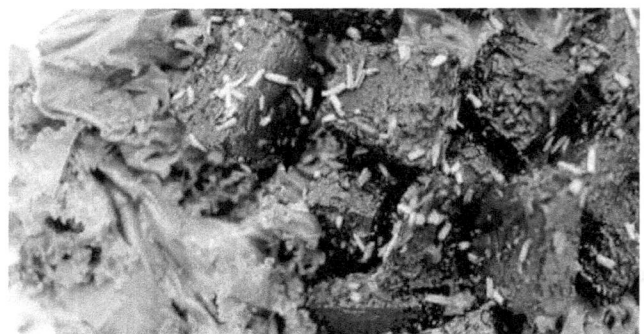

Ingredients

- 6 large leaves of kale (stalks omitted)
- 3 beets
- 1 tbsp minced garlic
- 1 tbsp extra virgin olive oil
- 1 tsp rosemary (or more, to taste)
- Sea salt and pepper, to taste
- This recipe makes 3 servings.

Instructions

- Preheat oven to 400 degrees Fahrenheit.
- Cut stalks and greens off of beets, then peel and chop into 1" cubes.
- Mix 1 tbsp olive oil, beet cubes, rosemary, sea salt, and pepper in a large bowl.
- Transfer beet mixture to baking dish and bake for 45 minutes, or until beets are tender enough to pierce with a fork.
- 10 minutes before the beets are ready, rip kale leaves into bite-size pieces.
- Add either a small amount of olive oil or water into a pan, and sauté kale and minced garlic on medium heat until wilted.
- Place kale onto a plate, and then add the beets on top.
- Serve and enjoy!!

Notes

- Calories: 123
- Total Fat: 5.4g
- Saturated Fat: 0.8g
- Carbs: 17.9g
- Fiber: 3.6g
- Protein: 4.1g

Kale and Red Pepper Frittata

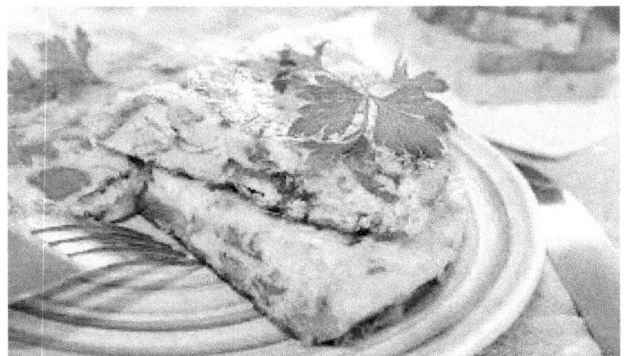

Ingredients

- 1 tbsp coconut oil
- 1/2 cup chopped red pepper
- 1/3 cup chopped onion
- 3 slices crispy bacon, chopped
- 2 cups chopped kale, de-stemmed and rinsed
- 8 large eggs
- 1/2 cup almond or coconut milk
- Salt and pepper to taste

Instructions

- Preheat oven to 350 degrees. In a medium bowl, whisk the eggs and milk together. Add salt and pepper. Set aside.
- In a non-stick skillet, heat about a tablespoon of coconut oil over medium heat. Add onion and red pepper and sauté for 3 minutes, until onion is translucent. Add kale and cook until it wilts, about 5 minutes.
- Add eggs to the pan mixture, along with the bacon. Cook for about 4 minutes until the bottom and edges of the frittata start to set.
- Put frittata in the oven and cook for 10-15 minutes until the frittata is cooked all the way through. Slice and serve.

Notes

- Servings: 4
- Difficulty: Easy

Paleo Chocolate Cookies (I Can't Get Enough of These)

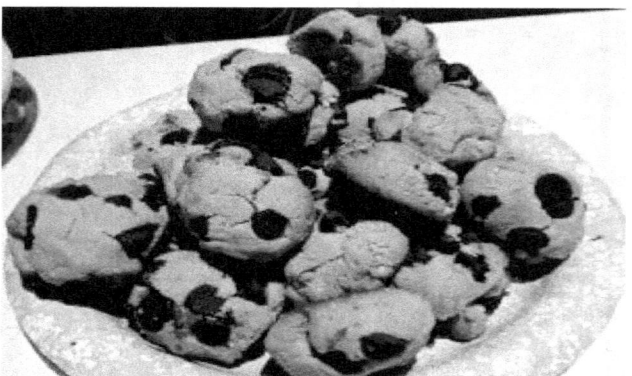

Ingredients

- 2 tbsp and 2 tsp coconut oil
- 3 oz. unsweetened dark chocolate

- 1/4 cup honey
- 2 eggs
- 1 1/2 tsp vanilla extract
- 1/2 cup coconut flour
- 1/2 tsp cinnamon

Instructions

- In a large microwave-safe bowl, melt the coconut oil and chocolate in the microwave, stirring intermittently. Let cool for 5 minutes.
- Add the eggs, vanilla, and honey to the chocolate mixture. Stir well to make sure not to scramble the eggs. Add in the coconut flour and cinnamon and mix well. Place in the refrigerator for approximately 30 minutes, until slightly hardened.
- Preheat oven to 350 degrees F. Roll out the dough between two pieces of parchment paper until 1/4-inch thick. Cut out shapes with a cookie cutter and carefully place on a parchment-lined baking sheet. Repeat this step for remaining dough.
- Bake cookies for 12-15 minutes. Allow to cool before serving.

Notes

- Servings: approximately 18 cookies
- Difficulty: Medium

Paleo French Toast with Blueberry Syrup

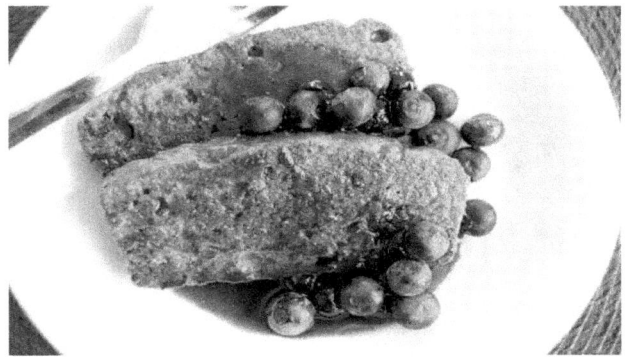

Ingredients

- 1 loaf Paleo bread (I used this recipe for Paleo Bread)
- 1/2 cup almond milk
- 2 eggs
- 1/2 tbsp vanilla
- 1 tsp cinnamon

Instructions

- In a large bowl, whisk together the coconut milk, eggs, vanilla and cinnamon.
- Heat a griddle or non-stick skillet to medium-high. Coat pan with coconut oil. Dip a slice of bread into the batter mixture to coat both sides, letting any excess drip off. Place the bread onto the pan and cook each side until slightly browned. Repeat with remaining bread. Serve warm.

Notes

- Servings: 4
- Difficulty: Easy

Lavender Maca Brownies (Dairy & Grain Free)

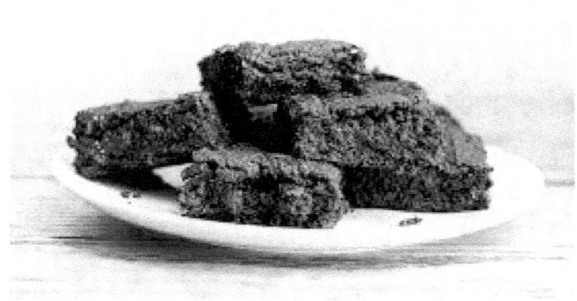

Ingredients

- 1/3 cup water
- 1/3 cup extra virgin olive oil
- 2 eggs
- 1 ½ cups almond flour
- 1 teaspoon baking powder
- 1 teaspoon salt
- 2/3 cup unsweetened cocoa powder
- 1 cup honey (I like to use raw honey found at my local farmer's market)
- ¾ cup semisweet chocolate chips
- 1 tablespoon dried lavender flowers (having a few left over for decoration)
- 1 tablespoon maca powder
- Himalayan pink salt (optional)

Directions

- Preheat oven to 350 degrees F and grease a 9x13" baking pan. (Brownies made in this size pan will be about one inch thick once baked – if you want them fuller, use a smaller sized pan)
- Whisk together the water, olive oil, and eggs in a large bowl.
- Slowly whisk in the flour, baking powder, salt, honey, maca powder, and cocoa powder one ingredient at a time. If you're using raw honey and it's too thick to whisk in, melt it in the microwave for about 20 seconds before adding it to your batter.
- Once the batter is well blended, add in your lavender and chocolate chips. The measurement for the lavender is up to you – I found one tablespoon to be the perfect amount, but depending on how floral you want these brownies to be you could add more or less.
- Pour the batter into a baking pan and spread until it is in one even layer. Don't worry if the batter seems too thick, that's how it's supposed to be.

- Bake for about 20 minutes, until a toothpick inserted in the center comes out clean.
- Let cool, then sprinkle fresh lavender and Himalayan pink salt over the top before cutting.
- Enjoy the fruits of your labor!!

Notes

1. This recipe should make approximately 24 2x2" square brownies.

Green Kale Smoothie with Mango

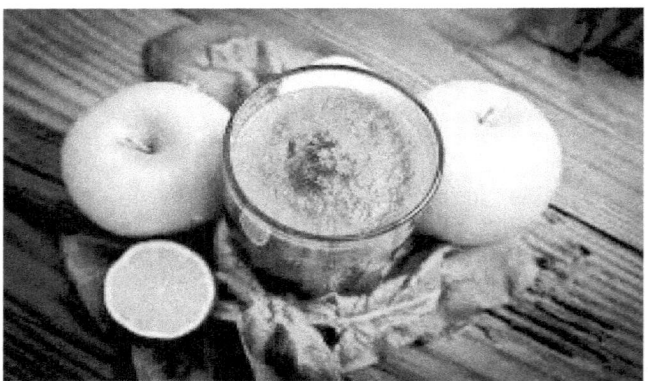

Ingredients

- 2 large leaves of kale
- 2 frozen bananas (peeled and cut into thirds)
- 1 frozen mango (diced)
- 2 tablespoons maca powder
- 2 tablespoons hemp hearts
- 3 cups unsweetened almond milk
- This recipe makes two large smoothies, can be halved for one serving.

Directions

- Add frozen banana chunks and frozen mango chunks into a blender with the almond milk. Blend until smooth. (I freeze my fruit in chunks to make it easier on the blender)
- Add in kale, maca powder, and hemp hearts. Blend until smooth.
- Serve immediately and enjoy!!

Nutrition Facts (per smoothie)

- Calories: 294
- Fat: 9.0g
- Saturated fat: 0.7g
- Sodium: 274mg
- Carbs: 51.0g
- Fiber: 8.6g
- Protein: 7.7g

Easy Paleo Shepherd's Pie

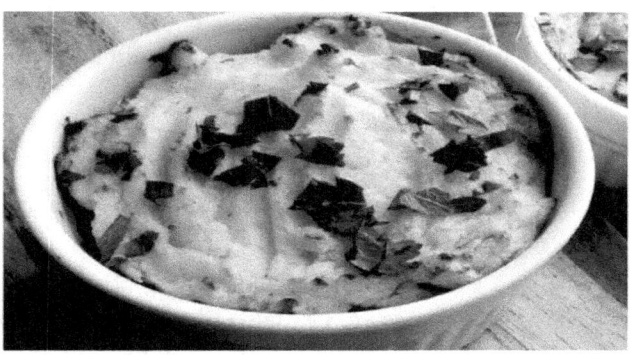

For the top layer

- 1 large head cauliflower, cut into florets
- 2 tbsp ghee, melted
- 1 tsp spicy Paleo mustard
- Salt and freshly ground black pepper, to taste
- Fresh parsley, to garnish

For the bottom layer

- 1 tbsp coconut oil
- 1/2 large onion, diced
- 3 carrots, diced
- 2 celery stalks, diced
- 1 lb. lean ground beef
- 2 tbsp tomato paste
- 1 cup chicken broth
- 1 tsp dry mustard
- 1/4 tsp cinnamon
- 1/8 tsp ground clove
- Salt and freshly ground black pepper, to taste

Instructions

- Place a couple inches of water in a large pot. Once the water is boiling, place steamer insert and then cauliflower florets into the pot and cover. Steam for 12-14 minutes, until tender. Drain and return cauliflower to the pot.
- Add the ghee, mustard, salt, and pepper to the cauliflower. Using an immersion blender or food processor, combine the ingredients until smooth. Set aside.
- Meanwhile, heat the coconut oil in a large skillet over medium heat. Add the onion, celery, and carrots and sauté for 5 minutes. Add in the ground beef and cook until browned.
- Stir the tomato paste, chicken broth, and remaining spices into the meat mixture. Season to taste with salt and pepper. Simmer until most of the liquid has evaporated, about 8 minutes, stirring occasionally.
- Distribute the meat mixture evenly among four ramekins and spread the pureed cauliflower on top. Use a fork to create texture in the cauliflower and drizzle with olive oil. Place under the broiler for 5-7 minutes until the top turns golden. Sprinkle with fresh parsley and serve.

Notes

- Servings: 4

- Difficulty: Medium

Spicy Avocado Dill Dressing

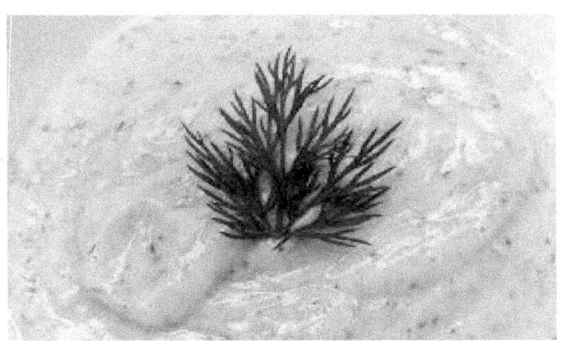

Ingredients

- 1 very ripe avocado
- 2 tablespoons olive oil
- 3 sprigs fresh dill
- 1 tbsp chili powder (more or less to taste)
- 1 tbsp lime juice
- 1 tbsp honey
- 2 tbsp apple cider vinegar
- 2 cloves garlic
- ¼ cup almond milk
- ¼ cup water

Directions

- Combine all ingredients in a blender, process until creamy.
- Store in an airtight jar or container in refrigerator, will last approximately 1 week.

Nutrition Facts per serving

- Calories: 104
- Fat: 9.2g
- Saturated Fat: 2.7g
- Carbs: 6.3g

- Fiber: 2.4g
- Protein: 1.1g

No-Bake Walnut Cookies (Grain-Free & Gluten-Free)

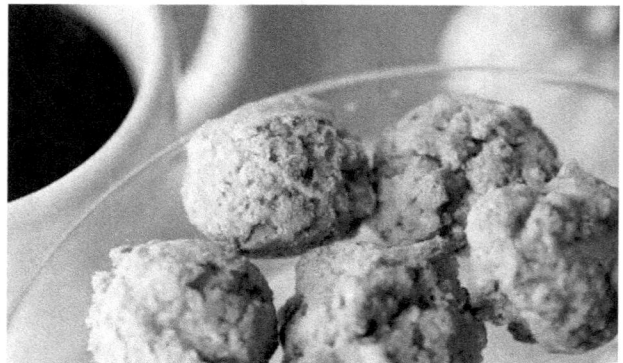

Ingredients

- 1 cup walnuts
- 1/2 cup unsweetened coconut flakes
- 2 tbsp raw honey
- 1/2 tsp vanilla extract
- 1/4 tsp salt

Directions

- Add walnuts to food processor and blend until finely ground. Add in the remaining ingredients and blend until a dough forms, about a minute.

- Turn out the dough onto a piece of parchment paper. Using your hands, roll pieces of the dough into small balls, about 1 inch around, and space out on parchment paper. After all of the balls are formed, press down on each ball to form a flat cookie. Place in the freezer for at least 30 minutes before serving. Store in an airtight container in the freezer.

Notes

- Servings: Makes 10-12 cookies
- Difficulty: Easy

Stove-top "Cheesy" Paleo Chicken Casserole

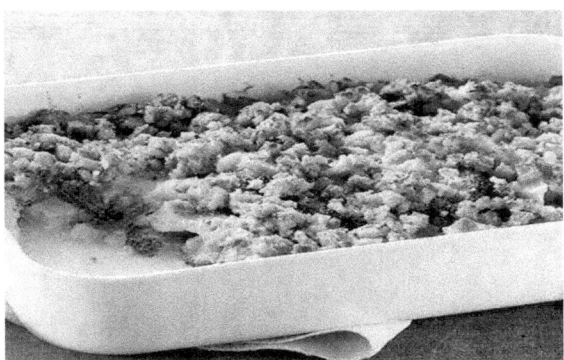

Ingredients

- 2 cups shredded cooked chicken
- 1 1/2 cups cooked butternut squash (about 1 small squash)
- 1/2 cup coconut cream, skimmed from the top of a can of coconut milk
- 1/4 cup coconut oil, melted
- 1 heaping cup green peas, thawed
- 1 tbsp apple cider vinegar
- 1/2 tsp salt

- 1/2 tsp oregano
- 1/2 tsp thyme
- 1 tbsp fresh parsley, for garnish

Instructions

- In a large bowl, mash the butternut squash. Stir in the coconut cream, oil, vinegar, salt, oregano, and thyme. Once everything is combined, add in the shredded chicken and peas.
- Place the mixture into a large saucepan and cook over medium heat for 5-8 minutes, until the peas are cooked and squash is creamy. Top with fresh parsley and serve warm.

Notes

- Servings: 4-5
- Difficulty: Medium

Legendary Gluten-Free Blueberry Crisp (YUM!)

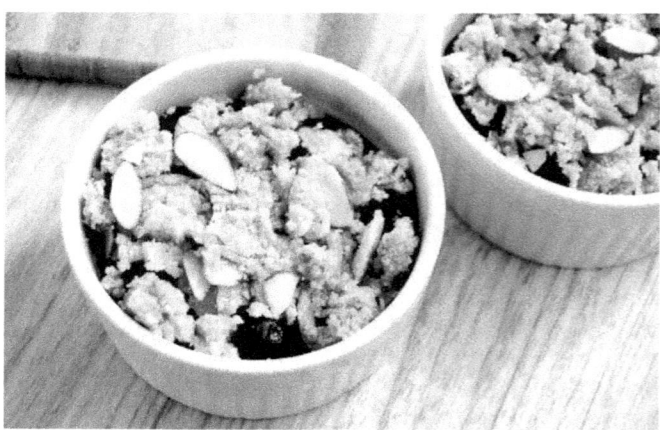

Ingredients

- 2 pints fresh blueberries
- Juice of 1 lemon
- 1 cup almond flour
- 1/2 cup slivered almonds
- 1/4 cup coconut oil, melted
- 2 tbsp maple syrup
- 1 tsp cinnamon
- 1/8 tsp salt
- Pinch of nutmeg

Instructions

- Preheat the oven to 375 degrees F. In a small bowl, toss the blueberries with the lemon juice. Divide between six ramekin dishes.
- Using the same bowl, mix together the remaining ingredients until combined. Spoon the almond crumble over the blueberries. Bake for 30-35 minutes, until bubbly and golden brown. Let cool slightly before serving.

Notes

1. Servings: 6 ramekins
2. Difficulty: Easy

Paleo Chicken Tortilla Soup

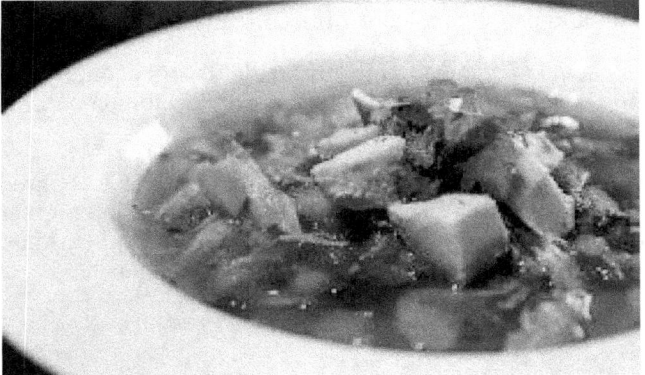

Ingredients

- 2 large chicken breasts, skin removed and cut into ½ inch strips
- 1 28oz can of diced tomatoes
- 32 ounces organic chicken broth
- 1 sweet onion, diced
- 2 jalepenos, de-seeded and diced
- 2 cups of shredded carrots
- 2 cups chopped celery
- 1 bunch of cilantro chopped fine
- 4 cloves of garlic, minced - I always use one of these
- 2 Tbs tomato paste
- 1 tsp chili powder
- 1 tsp cumin
- sea salt & fresh cracked pepper to taste

- olive oil
- 1-2 cups water

Instructions

- In a crockpot or large dutch oven over med-high heat, place a dash of olive oil and about ¼ cup chicken broth. Add onions, garlic, jalapeno, sea salt and pepper and cook until soft, adding more broth as needed.

- Then add all of your remaining ingredients and enough water to fill to the top of your pot. Cover and let cook on low for about 2 hrs, adjusting salt & pepper as needed.

- Once the chicken is fully cooked, you should be able to shred it very easily. I simply used the back of a wooden spoon and pressed the cooked chicken against the side of the pot. You could also use a fork or tongs to break the chicken apart and into shreds.

- Top with avocado slices and fresh cilantro. Enjoy!

- This is an easy one-pot meal that's loaded with veggies, low in fat, and full of flavor! You don't need to add cheese or tortilla strips the soup is full of flavor on it's own!

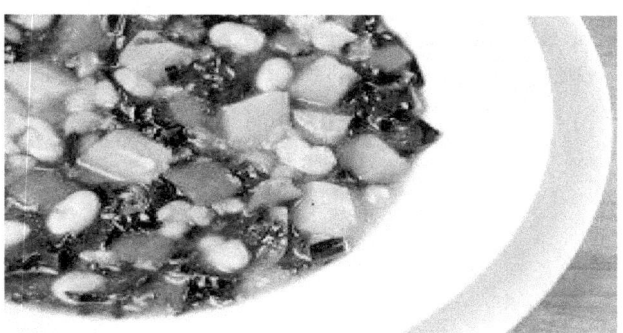

Ingredients:

- 2 tbsp bacon fat, or cooking oil of choice
- 2 lb stew beef, 1" cubed
- 1 onion, roughly chopped
- 4 garlic cloves, minced
- 1 1/2 tbsp fresh sage, minced
- 1/2 tsp smoked paprika
- 1 small butternut squash, cubed (about 4 cups)
- 16oz frozen, chopped kale (or one bunch fresh)
- 4 cups beef stock, preferably homemade
- salt and pepper

Instructions

- In a large dutch oven heat 1 tbsp bacon fat over medium high. Working in batches, brown the meat, making sure not to cook it through (it can turn tough). Set browned meat aside. Lower heat to medium and add the 2nd tbsp bacon fat. Once it's melted add the onions, garlic, smoked paprika, and sage to pot, along with a big pinch of salt and fresh pepper. Cook about 8 minutes, or until the onions begin to soften and turn translucent. Make sure to stir frequently so the mixture doesn't burn.

- Add the beef, butternut squash, and kale to the pot. Stir to combine, then add the chicken stock and two cups of hot water. Bring to a boil, then reduce to a simmer and let cook, covered, for at least an hour. I let mine go about 45 minutes longer.

Bacon and Tomato Quiche

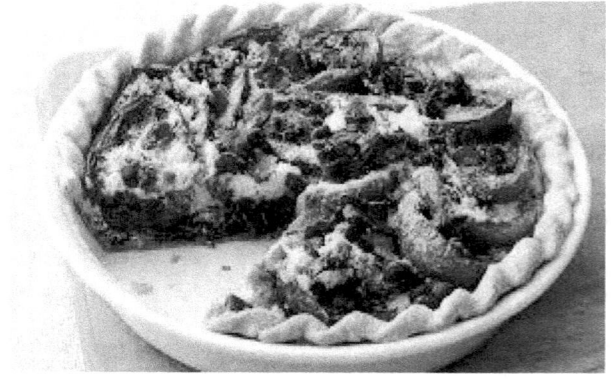

Ingredients

Zucchini Hash Crust:

- 2 small to medium size organic zucchini, grated
- 1 egg, beaten
- 1 1/2 Tbsp coconut flour
- 1 tsp flax meal *optional
- 1 tbsp butter or coconut oil melted
- 1/8 tsp sea salt

Quiche:
- 5 eggs, beaten
- 1/2 cup organic egg whites, (I used the ones in a carton, but make sure egg white is the only ingredient) or you could separate 3 eggs
- 3 Tbsp milk of choice: organic heavy cream, or unsweetened plain almond milk
- 5 slices nitrate free bacon, cooked and chopped (make sure bacon has no sugar in the ingredients)
- 2/3 cup cauliflower, ground into rice (you won't taste it, and it adds nutrients and fiber)
- 1/2 cup fresh spinach, chopped * optional
- 1/4 tsp ground mustard
- 1/4 tsp sea salt (I use Real Salt or Himalayan sea salt)
- 1/4 tsp black pepper

Topping:
- 2 small to medium sized tomatoes, sliced (I used 6 slices).
- 1/2 cup grated cheese of choice * optional

Instructions

- Preheat oven to 400 F, and grease or oil pie dish.
- Grate or use processor on zucchini.
- Wrap grated zucchini in layered paper towels or cheese cloth. Squeeze and drain liquid from zucchini over sink. Place drained zucchini in large bowl.
- Add all the remaining crust ingredients to the zucchini and mix together.

- Place zucchini mixture into pie dish. Use the back of a spoon to spread mixture around pie dish, until dish is covered in zucchini crust mixture.
- Bake zucchini crust in oven for 9 minutes.
- Remove crust from oven (leave oven on). Set aside.
- In large mixing bowl combine: eggs, egg whites, milk of choice, ground mustard, sea salt, and black pepper.
- Grate or use processor on the cauliflower until rice texture forms.
- Add cauliflower rice, chopped spinach, and chopped bacon to the egg mixture and combine.
- Pour egg mixture into zucchini crust.
- Place tomato slices on top of quiche.
- Bake for 28 minutes, but check at 20 minutes to see if crust edges are browning too much.
- Loosely cover the top of pie dish with a parchment paper sheet. Place back in oven for remaining 8 minutes, or until top is browned and center is firm and set.
- Add optional cheese and put back in oven for 2 minutes.
- Remove and let cool.
- Slice and serve.

Notes

- Net Carb Count*: 8.15 g net carbs (per 1 slice - makes 8 slices)
- Total Carb Count: 11.79 g total carbs (per 1 slice - makes 8 slices)

DINNER

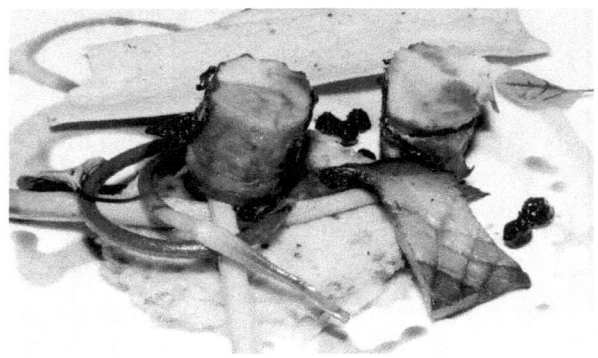

Yields: 12 total strawberries/baby bell peppers

- 6 strawberries
- 6 golden baby bell peppers
- Honey Basil Ricotta (see below)
- 1 oz. thinly sliced grass-fed proscuitto, divided into 12 strips
- 1/4 c. micro greens (about half a small package)

Instructions

- Using a sharp pairing knife, cut the tops off the strawberries, pulling the middle completely out and leaving a deep hole. Do the same for the peppers and use your finger to pull any seeds out of the insides.
- To assemble: use a butter knife to stuff the berries/peppers with about 1 t. each of the Honey Basil Ricotta (the peppers will hold more ricotta than the berries). Then place a few sprigs of micro greens into the ricotta. Wrap a thin slice of proscuitto around each one and lay down length-wise to hold the proscuitto in place (you could also use toothpicks for this but that's a little too fussy for me).

Vanilla Pumpkin Seed Clusters

Ingredients:

- 115g (1/2 cup) pumpkin seeds
- 1 tsp vanilla extract
- 2 tsp honey
- 2 tsp coconut sugar
- Water (boiled)

Instructions

- Preheat oven to 150c.
- In a medium bowl, combine the honey, coconut sugar and vanilla. Stir together to create a thick paste then add a small drop of boiled water to thin it out and create a runny syrup.
- Pour in the pumpkin seeds and stir them around in the mixture to evenly coat them.
- Dollop a generous tsp full of the pumpkin seeds onto a baking sheet, repeat until it's all used up and cook for 15-20 minutes until most of the seeds have browned (but don't let them burn!)
- Take out of the oven and leave to cool for a few minutes. Once they've cooled a little (but are still warm) you can press the clusters together to make sure they don't fall apart. They will dry quickly.
- Once they're cooled and dried, they're ready to eat! Enjoy on their own or served on top of your cereal.

Almond Joy Sunday

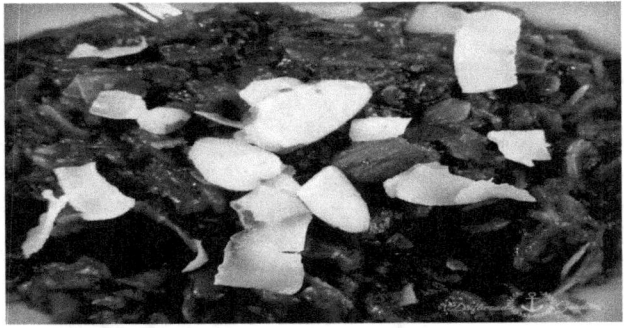

Ingredients:

1. 2 cans full fat coconut milk
- ½ cup honey
- 1 ½ tablespoons vanilla extract
- 1 dark baking chocolate bar
- ¼ cup sliced almonds
- ½ cup unsweetened coconut flakes

Instructions

- In a blender,mix together the coconut milk, honey, and vanilla extract. Line a plastic Tupperware with plastic wrap. Pour the mixture into it and freeze it overnight. The next day, take half of the frozen mixture and add it to a food processor. Mix it on high until it resembles frozen yogurt and put it back into a storage container. Repeat this process with the other half of the mixture. Return the blended ice cream to the freeze for 30 minutes before serving.

2. To assemble, melt the chocolate chips in a saucepan over low heat, to prevent burning the chocolate. Serve each Almond Joy Sunday with a scoop of the ice cream. Drizzle the melted chocolate on top, then sprinkle with coconut flakes and sliced almonds. Serve immediately.

Spiced
Apples
Brandy

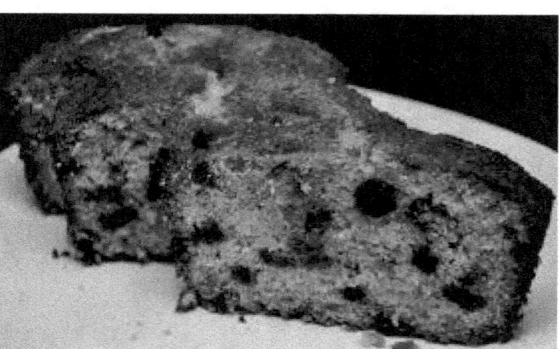

Autumn
Baked in

Ingredients

- 2 apples of your choice (I used gala, but choose your favorite!)
- 1 cup brandy
- 1/4 cup walnuts
- 1/4 cup raisins
- 1/4 tablespoon nutmeg
- 1/4 tablespoon cinnamon
- 1/4 tablespoon ground cloves

Directions

- Preheat oven to 350 degrees Fahrenheit.
- Slice the very top and very bottom off of each apple. (The top allows for more room to stuff with goodies, the bottom allows the apples to soak up all the nice sauce).
- Core both apples to the bottom, but not all the way through.
- Mix brandy, spices, walnuts, and raisins in a small bowl.
- Pour half of the brandy spice mixture into each apple.
- Place on baking sheet and bake 20-25 minutes, or until apples are soft. I like to pour any remaining sauce mixture into the bottom of the pan so the apples can soak up the flavors.
- Serve and enjoy! My roommate enjoyed his with a side of vanilla coconut milk ice cream.

Notes

Recipe makes 2 servings

Nutrition Facts Per Serving

- Calories: 353
- Total Fat: 10.0g
- Saturated Fat: 0.6g
- Carbs: 32.4g
- Fiber: 4.0g
- Protein: 4.6g

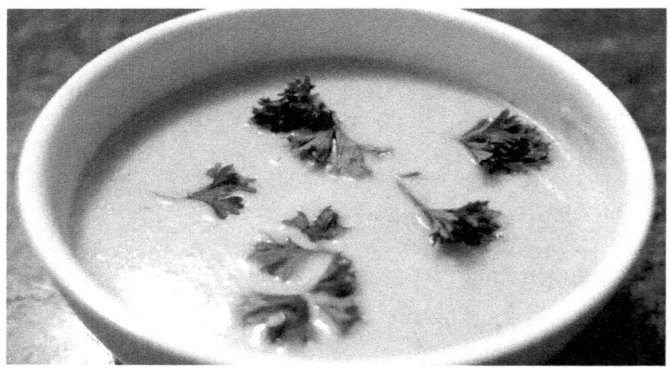

Ingredients

- 2 tbsp olive oil
- 1 onion, chopped
- 1 large head of cauliflower, cut into florets
- 3 cups low-sodium chicken stock
- 1/2 tsp coriander
- 1/2 tsp turmeric
- 1 1/2 tsp cumin
- 1 cup full-fat coconut milk
- 1/4 cup roasted cashews
- 2 tbsp fresh parsley, finely chopped
- Salt and pepper, to taste

Instructions

- Preheat the oven to 375 degrees F. Spread out the onion and cauliflower in a single layer on a baking sheet. Drizzle with olive oil and sprinkle with salt and pepper. Roast for 15-20 minutes until golden, stirring once.
- Place the cauliflower and onions in a large pot and add the chicken stock. Stir in the coriander, turmeric, cumin, and a pinch of salt. Bring to a boil and let boil for 5 minutes. Remove from heat.

- Using an immersion blender, puree ingredients in the pot until smooth. (Alternatively, carefully transfer to a blender.) Stir in the coconut milk and warm the soup to serve. Taste to adjust seasonings as necessary. Serve with roasted cashews and top with parsley.

Notes

- Servings: 3-4
- Difficulty: Easy

Fresh and Easy Arugula Pesto

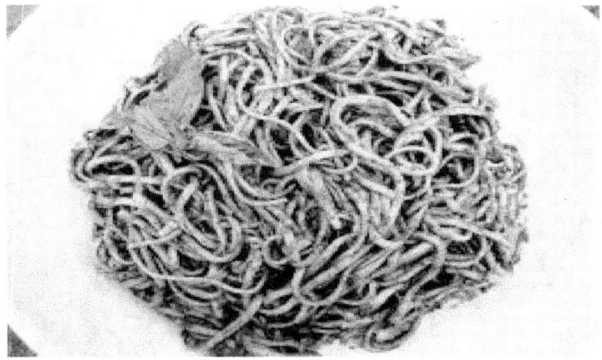

Ingredients

- 2 cups fresh arugula, packed
- 1/4 cup walnuts
- 2 cloves garlic, peeled
- 1/2 tsp lemon juice
- 1/2 tsp salt
- 1/2 cup extra virgin olive oil

Instructions

- Add the arugula, walnuts, garlic, lemon juice, and salt to a blender or food processor and blend. Gradually add the olive oil and process until well combined.

Notes

- Servings: about 2/3 cup
- Difficulty: Easy

Homemade Paleo BBQ Sauce (YUM)

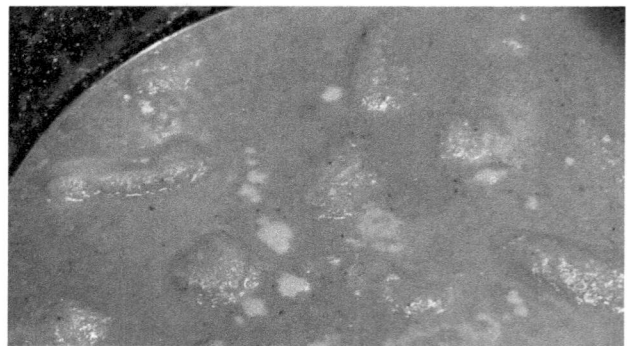

Ingredients

- 15 oz. organic tomato sauce
- 1 cup water
- 1/2 cup apple cider vinegar
- 1/3 cup honey
- 1 tbsp lemon juice

- 2 tsp onion powder
- 1 1/2 tsp ground black pepper
- 1 1/2 tsp ground mustard
- 1 tsp paprika

Instructions

- Combine all of the ingredients in a medium saucepan over medium-high heat. Stir to combine. Bring to a boil, and then reduce to simmer for 1 hour. Taste and adjust seasonings as desired. Serve with meat or store in an airtight container in the refrigerator.

Notes

- Servings: about 1 1/2 cups
- Difficulty: Easy

Basil Pesto

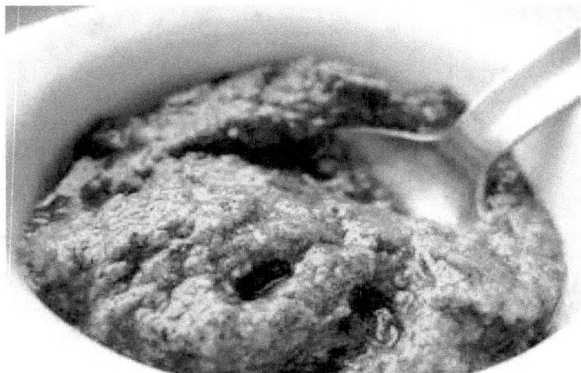

Ingredients
- 1 large bunch of basil (approx. 2 cups)
- 1/3 cup walnuts or pine nuts

- 2 medium garlic cloves, minced
- 1/2 cup Parmigiano Reggiano or other Parmesan cheese (optional)
- approx. 1/3 cup extra virgin olive oil
- salt and pepper to taste

Instructions

- Place basil, nuts, garlic and cheese (optional) in food processor.

- Run the food processor, pausing to add olive oil to reach desired consistency.

- 3) Salt and pepper to taste.

Radicchio Pesto

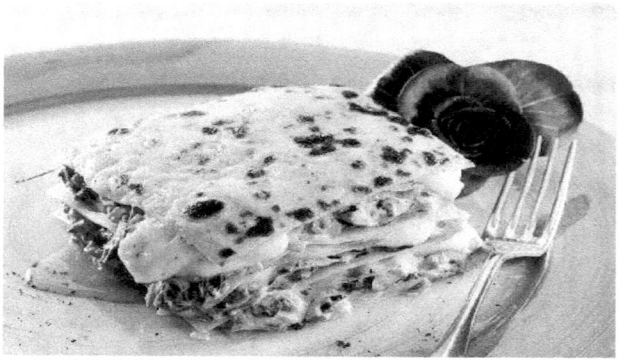

- **Ingredients**
  Serves 4

  1. 1 radicchio head, roughly chopped (ribs and leaves)
  2. 3 tablespoons grated Romano cheese
  3. 3 tablespoons grated Parmesan cheese

4. ⅓ cup / 1.8 oz / 50 gr blanched almonds
5. 5 tablespoons warm water, plus more if needed
6. ½ teaspoon fine grain sea salt
7. Ground black pepper to taste
8. 2 tablespoons olive oil

Directions

1. Place the cut radicchio in a small bowl of cold water and allow to sit for 30 minutes. This will remove some of the bitterness. Drain and squeeze out as much water as possible. (Note: you can skip this step if you're in a hurry).
2. Heat a skillet over medium heat. Add almonds and toast for 5 minutes. Set aside.
3. In a food processor add (toasted) almonds; pulse until the mixture resembles a coarse meal. Add the radicchio and 2 tablespoons of water.
4. Pulse until the radicchio is broken up and nearly smooth.
5. Using a spatula, scrape down the sides.
6. Add Parmesan cheese, Romano cheese, salt and pepper. Pulse again and while the food processor is running slowly add the water - one tablespoon at a time - until the pesto reaches a creamy consistency.
7. Transfer radicchio pesto to a bowl and using a spoon stir in the olive oil until it's completely absorbed.

8. If the pesto looks too thick, add more olive oil (or water), one tablespoon   at a time until it reaches the desired consistency.

Nutrition facts

One serving yields 165 calories, 15 grams of fat, 3 grams of carbs and 6 grams of protein

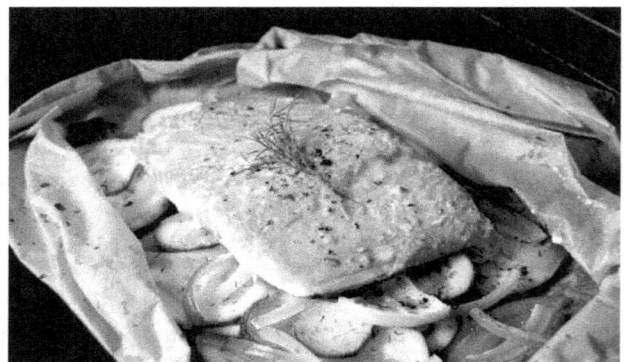

Ingredients

- 2 6-oz. salmon fillets
- 2 zucchini, halved lengthwise and thinly sliced
- 1/4 red onion, thinly sliced
- 1 tsp fresh dill, chopped
- 2 slices lemon
- 1 tbsp fresh lemon juice
- Extra virgin olive oil, for drizzling
- Salt and freshly ground pepper

Instructions

- Preheat the oven to 350 degrees F. Prepare two large pieces of parchment paper by folding them in half to crease. Then open the papers and lay flat.
- On one side of the crease, place half of the zucchini, red onion, dill, and one lemon slice. Drizzle with olive oil and sprinkle with salt and pepper. Place a salmon fillet on top and drizzle with the lemon juice. Season with salt and pepper. Repeat with the second piece of parchment paper and remaining ingredients.

- Fold the parchment paper over the salmon to close, making a half-moon shape. Seal the open sides by folding small pleats in the paper. Place the parchment packets on a rimmed baking sheet and bake for 15-20 minutes until the salmon is opaque. Serve warm.

Notes

- Servings: 2
- Difficulty: Medium

Healthy Low Carb Crustless Quiche Recipe

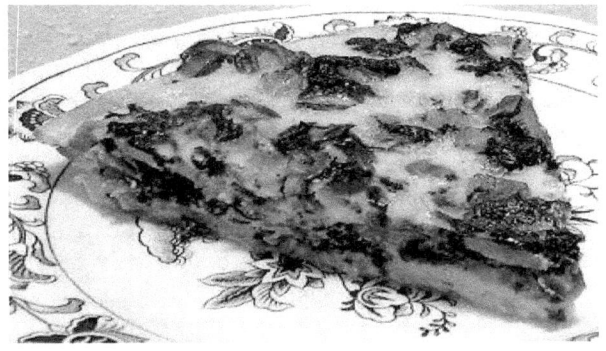

- 6 organic, free range eggs

- 6 stalks kale

- 6 stalks swiss chard

- 15 campari tomatoes, 10 cut into quarters and 5 with stem attached

- 2 medium shallots sliced thin, or half a sweet onion, diced

- 1 Tbs whole grain mustard

- 1 tsp garlic powder

- 1/4 tsp red pepper flakes – use more or less to taste
- 4 oz shredded parmesan cheese
- 1 Tbs organic butter
- salt and pepper

Instructions

- Preheat your oven to 350 degrees F (175 degrees C).
- In a <u>nonstick skillet</u> over med-high heat, melt your butter. Add shallots and a little salt and pepper and cook until translucent, about 2 mins.
- Grab your kale and swiss chard by the stem and strip the leaves from the stem with your hands. (I like to save the stems and use them later in my veggie juices)! Again, using your hands, tear the leaves into small pieces and add to your skillet. Next add your tomatoes, mustard, red pepper flakes, and more salt & pepper. Using a <u>wooden spoon</u>, stir all ingredients together, taste and adjust spices as needed, and remove from heat.
- Whisk eggs and parmesan in a large bowl until well combined. Pour the egg mixture into your skillet and stir to combine with the vegetables. Then top with your tomatoes on the vine. You could also transfer all of your ingredients into a <u>baking or pie dish</u>, but I like to keep it simple so I bake the dish in the same skillet; just remember to use an <u>oven mitt</u> to remove from the oven!
- Bake until golden brown and eggs are completely set, about 30- 35 mins. Allow quiche to cool for 10 minutes before serving.

Sun-Dried Tomato Quiche

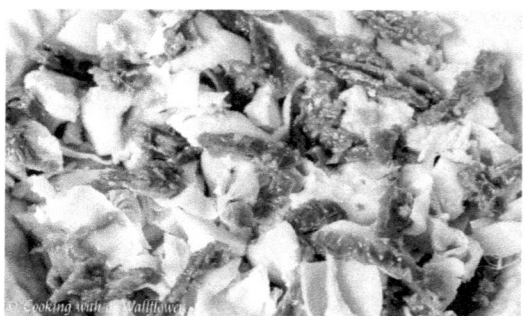

INGREDIENTS

- 5 eggs
- 1 zucchini
- 1 onion
- ¼ tsp salt
- ¼ tsp pepper
- 2 tsp coconut oil
- 2 tomatoes, small
- 4 oz sundried tomatoes
- ¼ lb pancetta, sliced

INSTRUCTIONS

- Preheat oven to 350° F.
- Grease an 8-inch cast-iron skillet with 1 tsp coconut oil and set aside.
- Melt 1 tsp coconut oil in a medium skillet over medium heat. Whirl the onion and zucchini in a food processor until finely shredded, then cook in the skillet until soft and translucent, about 10 minutes.
- While the zucchini and onions soften, drain the oil from your sun-dried tomatoes if you're using oil-packed. Roughly chop and add to a medium mixing bowl.
- Pull the pancetta slices apart with your fingers into shreds, then add to the tomatoes.
- When the onions and zucchini are soft, add to the pancetta and tomatoes. Mix thoroughly and allow to cool to room temperature. Whisk in eggs, salt and pepper and pour into the cast-iron skillet.
- Cook in the preheated oven for 1 hour and 15 minutes or until firm.
- Serve warm.

Asparagus Quiche with Spaghetti Squash Crust

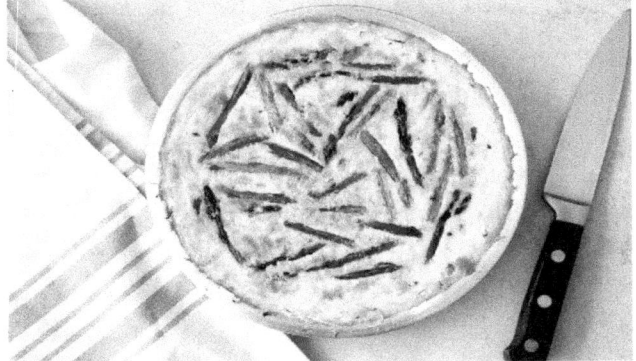

Ingredients

- 1 medium spaghetti squash (use about 2 1/2 – 3 cups of the meat for this recipe)
- 2 tablespoons butter
- 1 large leek, thinly sliced
- 3 tablespoons butter
- 5 large eggs, beaten
- 1 cup coconut milk/almond milk/dairy milk (I used almond milk, as that's all that we had left)
- a bunch of thin asparagus (about 2 cups), cut in halves or large pieces
- 1 medium tomato, cut in thin slices and then halve the slices
- sea salt and freshly ground pepper, to taste
- 1/2 – 1 teaspoon ground nutmeg

Instructions

- Preheat the oven to 375F (190C).
- Carefully split the spaghetti squash in half. (It can also be baked whole, but it will take longer.)
- Remove the seeds and sprouts, if any, with hands.
- Place cut-side down on a baking pan.
- Bake for 40 minutes, or until tender.
- In the meantime, poach the asparagus in some water, until just tender. Remove from water and set aside.
- Allow the spaghetti squash to cool a bit before removing the meat with a fork.

- Mix about 2 1/2 to 3 cups of the meat with 2 tablespoons of butter and mix well.
- Add sea salt and pepper, to taste. (Remember that the egg mixture will also contain seasoning, so don't go overboard.)
- Pat the squash into a quiche form, covering the sides and bottom.
- Bake at 400F (200C) for about 5-8 minutes, until golden and slightly crispy. Remove from oven and set aside.
- In a saucepan, over medium heat, cook the leek slices with the 3 tablespoons butter, until tender.
- Allow to slightly cool before pouring into the beaten eggs.
- Add the milk, nutmeg, sea salt and pepper to taste.
- Place the poached asparagus pieces on top of the spaghetti squash crust.
- Pour the beaten eggs and leeks over top, covering the asparagus evenly.
- Place the tomato pieces on top.
- Bake for 35-40 minutes.

Coconut Crust Quiche

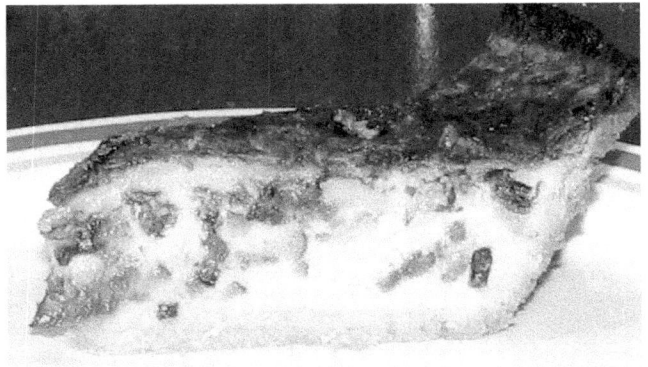

- **Ingredients crust:**

  1 cup of coconut flour (about 140 grams)
  3 eggs
  pinch of salt
- 1/4 tsp garlic powder
  1/4 tsp chili powder
  black pepper
  1/4 cup butter, soft (or ghee)
  2 tbsp water
  2 tbsp coconut oil, melted

  Mix all of the ingredients together, the dough will be a bit dry and crumbly. Line a springform pan with the dough (I used a pan that is 20cm in diameter)

  Instructions

  In a bowl, mix your favorite quiche ingredients together: [not all paleo]

- 8 eggs
  1 onion, chopped & cooked
  dried chives
  2 tomatoes, chopped
  pepper
  [1/2 cup shredded cheese]
  bacon, chopped
  pinch of salt
  Simply pour the mix in the pan, and bake in the oven on 180C (350F) for about 45 mins.

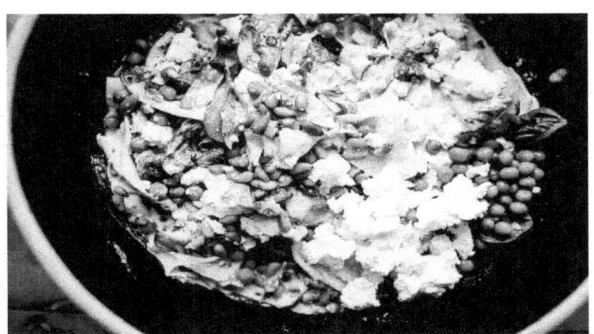

Garden Pea, Feta & Mint Tart (serves 6-8)
Crust:

- 1/2 cup butter, melted
- 2 large eggs
- 3/4 cup coconut flour
- 1/2 tsp sea salt

Instruction
- Whisk together the eggs and butter.
- Sieve the coconut flour into a large mixing bowl. Add the salt.
- Gradually add the wet ingredients to the dry and mix until it forms a soft batter.
- Press this into a greased 9in pie dish. It won't cooperate like regular dough, that's ok. Just press it in with your hands until the dish is covered. Prick the base.
- Bake at 375 for 5 minutes. Remove and let cool while you sort out the filling.

Filling:

- 4oz feta cheese, crumbled
- 1 1/2 cups peas (I used frozen and defrosted beforehand)

- 2 spring/green onions, finely chopped
- 2 tbsps fresh mint leaves, chopped
- 3 large eggs
- 1/2 cup plain yoghurt
- salt and pepper

Instructions

- Whisk the eggs, yoghurt and seasoning together. Stir in the peas, feta and onions.
- Fold in the mint and pour the whole mixture into your pie crust.
- Bake at 375 for 25-30 mins til firm. Let cool for a few minutes before slicing up.

Garlicky Collard Pie

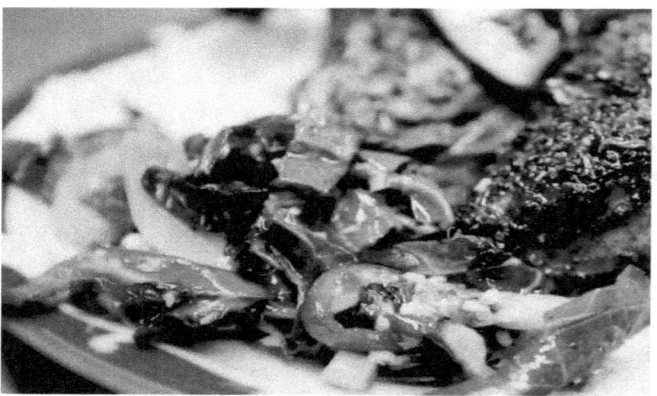

Ingredients

- 2 tablespoons ghee, butter or lard
- 1 small yellow onion, diced
- 4 cloves garlic, minced
- 4 cups collards or other hearty greens, rinsed and chopped
- 1 1/2 teaspoons kosher or sea salt
- 3/4 teaspoon freshly-ground black pepper

- 2 ounces pecorino romano or other hard Italian cheese, shredded
- 10 large eggs
- 3/4 cup coconut milk plus 1/2 cup water or 1 1/4 cups half and half
- 2 teaspoons garlic powder
- 1 teaspoon dried thyme
- 1 teaspoon dried oregano

Instructions

- Preheat the oven to 375 F. Generously grease a 10" deep-dish pie plate with butter or non-hydrogenated palm oil shortening.
- Melt the ghee in a large, heavy skillet over medium heat. Cook the onion until soft and almost translucent, about 5 minutes; add the garlic and cook for another minute more. Add the collard greens and cook, stirring frequently, until they are wilted. Season with the salt and pepper and remove from the heat.
- In a large bowl, whisk together the eggs with the water, coconut milk, garlic powder, thyme and oregano until well blended. Spread the collard/onion mixture over the bottom of the greased pie plate; sprinkle the cheese evenly over the greens. Carefully pour the egg mixture over the cheese and greens.
- Bake the pie for 25 to 35 minutes, or until the top is golden brown and a knife inserted in the center comes out clean.
- Cool for 30 minutes before cutting into wedges. Serve with a chunky salsa or warm marinara sauce.
- Nutrition (per serving): 203 calories, 15.5g total fat, 247.5mg cholesterol, 534.7mg sodium, 210.4mg potassium, 5.2g carbohydrates, 1.1g fiber, <1g sugar, 11.3g protein.

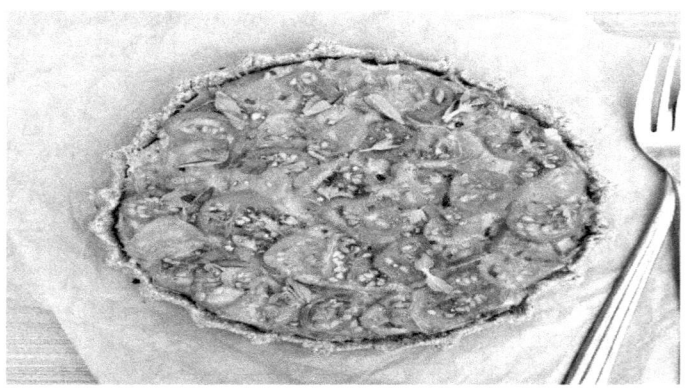

1. 1 medium onion, chopped
2. 1 pound of bulk sausage (just remove casings if you can't find it in bulk)
3. 2 cloves of garlic, grated
4. coconut oil
5. 12 oz. of broccoli
6. 10 eggs
7. sea salt/pepper/TJ's 21 seasoning salute

Instructions:

- Preheat your oven to 350 degrees. saute the onion in coconut oil over medium-high*ish* heat. season with salt, pepper and 21 salute. once the onions are cooked halfway (translucent and soft) add the sausage meat. crumble the sausage as it cooks.

- As the sausage is cooking, liberally grease a 9 x 13 pan in coconut oil. i suggest a small sandwich bag over your hand so you don't miss any spots or corners. next, in a large bowl, whisk the eggs vigorously. season with salt and pepper.

- The broccoli i used was frozen in one of the steam-ready bags you throw into the microwave. instead of cooking it for 5 minutes in the microwave, i cooked it for only 2 so it was defrosted but not cooked all the way through. if you are using fresh broccoli, i would suggest blanching it for a minute or 2, any longer than that and it might get mushy. add the broccoli to the sausage mixture and cook for a minute or two.

- Finally, add the garlic to the sausage mixture, cook for one additional minute and then remove from the heat. place the broccoli-sausage mixture into the greased baking dish. pour the eggs over the top of the meat and vegetables and bake uncovered for 25-30 minutes.

Crustless Mini Quiches

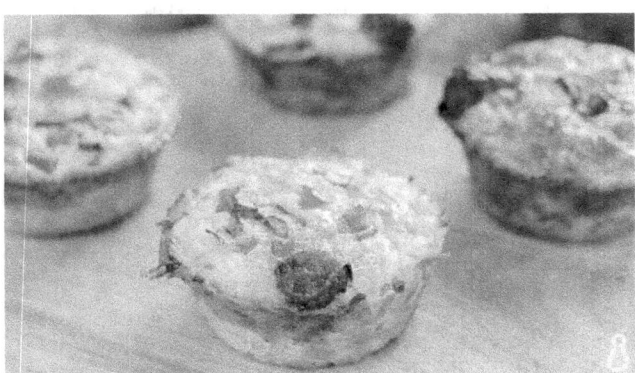

Ingredients

- 12 Large Omega 3 or other cage free, vegetarian fed, etc eggs
  8 slices of bacon chopped and precooked

- 1 large carrot grated
- 1 large handful of spinach chopped finely
- 3 mini red bell peppers (or a couple tablespoons of a whole one), diced
- 3 mini yellow bell peppers (or part of a large one), diced
- 1/2 cup of chopped broccoli florets
- 2 green onions (or more if you like a strong onion flavor), chopped finely

- 1 chicken breast precooked with salt and pepper, diced (or any leftover meat, I just had this in the fridge)

Instructions

- Preheat your oven to 350 degrees. Combine all of your ingredients and beat on high till frothy with electric mixer. Grease muffin tins with coconut oil liberally and pour in mixture 1/4 per muffin cup.

- Making sure to keep stirring up those goodies so they don't sink to the bottom while your filling your muffin cups. Bake at 350 degrees for about 20-25 minutes depending on your oven and muffin pans.

- Remove from oven and allow to cool for a few minutes, then run a knife around the edges to loosen, remove and eat warm or allow to cool completely to store for later.

- These are a great grab and go breakfast or post WOD snack, make them ahead on the weekend and just warm up in the morning and go.

- Post comments on your favorite versions to share with others. We would love to hear from you.

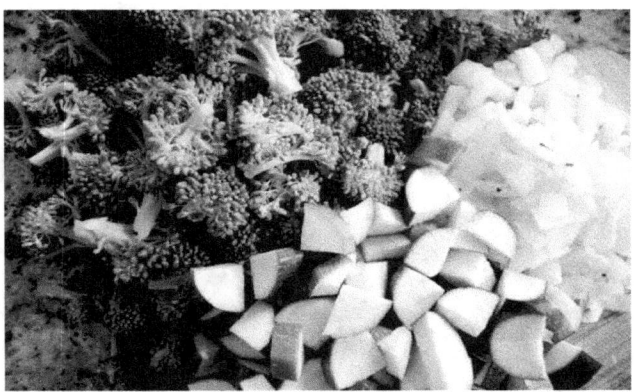

Ingredients

- 8 eggs
- 1/2 large onion, diced
- 2 medium zucchini, diced
- 1 medium head of broccoli, chopped
- 1 tsp salt
- 1/2 tsp freshly ground black pepper
- 1 tbsp fresh parsley, chopped

Instructions

- Preheat the oven to 350 degrees F. In a small bowl, whisk the eggs, salt and pepper. Stir in the chopped vegetables.
- Grease a ramekin with coconut oil spray. Pour egg mixture into the dish and bake for 25-30 minutes or until the eggs are set. Remove from heat and let sit for 5 minutes before serving. Top with chopped parsley to serve.

Notes

- Servings: 6
- Difficulty: Easy

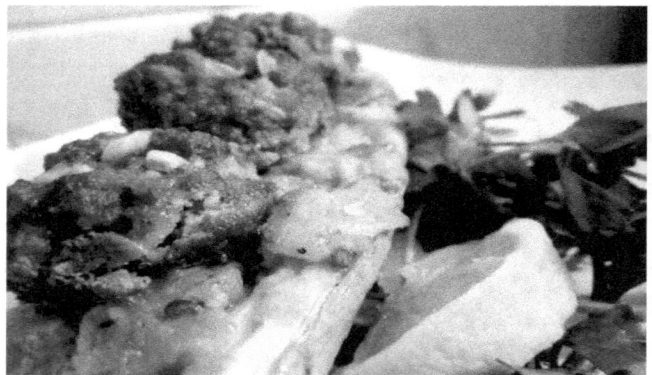

Meatballs

- ½ onion
- ½ tomato
- 4 cloves of garlic
- 1 egg
- 2 tbsp coconut milk
- 2 tsp sea salt
- ½ tsp black pepper
- ½ tsp paprika
- 1 lb. of grass-fed ground beef.

Zucchini "bread" and coconut sauce

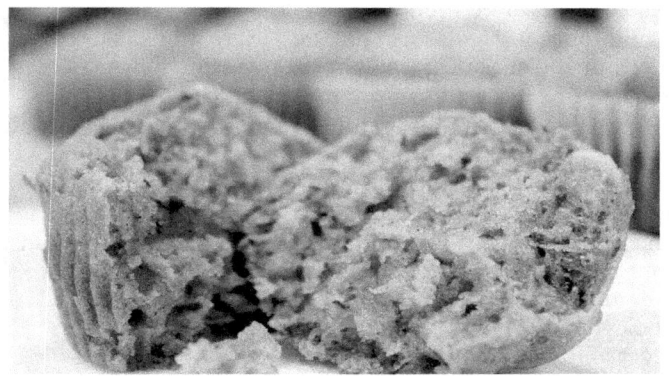

- 1 onion
- 1 tomato
- 3 cloves of garlic
- 250g can coconut milk
- 4 very large zucchinis or 8 small ones (one per sandwich)
- 1 tsp sea salt
- 1 tsp curry powder
- 1 lemon
- Parsley

Instructions

- Preheat your over to 350 degrees. Line two roasting trays with aluminum foil.
- Dice your tomato, onion and garlic. Set aside.
- For the meatballs, crack open your egg and mix in tomato, onion, garlic, salt, black pepper and coconut milk.
- It's time to get intimate with your creation. Put your beef into a mixing bowl and using your hands knead in the egg mixture. Shape

into lovely little meatballs and place on roasting tray and put tray into heated oven for 20 minutes.

- While your meatballs form into edible creations take your washed zucchini and slice them in half. Then dig out about 1/3 of the zucchini meat on one half and ½ from the top half.
- Dice up the zucchini meat and add onion, tomato, garlic, salt, curry powder and add the coconut cream only (the water on the bottom is not needed so use it tomorrow for a tasty addition to a Crockpot chicken soup).
- Mix everything and pour into your waiting zucchini tunnels. Remove your meatballs from the oven and place your zucchini into the oven at the same temperature.
- Cook your guys for 20 minutes uncovered and then cover them with a sheet of foil for another 10 minutes.
- Chop up your parsley and lemon wedges for plating.
- Remove zucchini from oven and sprinkle some lemon juice on top. Nestle the meatballs into the deeper zucchini half place your second zucchini half on top, slice in half and serve with some parsley and lemon on the side for a mini salad garnish.

Notes

- You can use a knife and fork but for sandwich-style eating wrap the bottom halves of your sandwiches in wax paper (the red and white checkered kind if you can get it) so you can hold on to your grub and have a delightful conversation at the same time.

Vegetarian Thai Red Curry with Squash

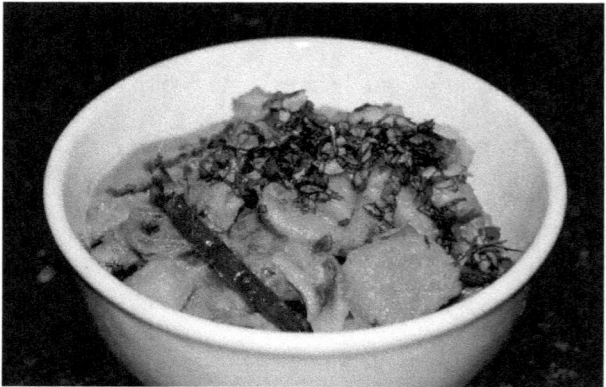

Ingredients

- 1 tbsp coconut oil
- 1 medium yellow onion, diced
- 1 tsp salt
- 1 green bell pepper, thinly sliced
- 4 cloves garlic, minced
- 1-inch piece fresh ginger, peeled and minced
- 3 tbsp Thai red curry paste
- 1 14-oz. can coconut milk
- 1 tbsp coconut aminos
- 1 large acorn squash, peeled, seeded, and cut into 1-inch cubes
- 2 tsp lime juice
- 1/4 cup cilantro, chopped
- Cauliflower rice, for serving

Instructions

- Melt the coconut oil in a large pan over medium heat. Add the onion and cook for 5-6 minutes, stirring occasionally. Add the bell pepper, garlic, ginger, and salt and stir to combine. Cook for an additional minute.
- Add the curry paste to the pan and cook for about a minute, stirring to coat the other ingredients. Add in the coconut milk and coconut aminos and bring to a simmer. Stir in the squash. Simmer, stirring occasionally, for 15-20 minutes until the squash is fork-tender. Remove the pan from the heat and stir in the lime juice. Taste and adjust salt and lime juice as necessary. Sprinkle with cilantro to serve.

Notes

- Servings: 4
- Difficulty: Medium

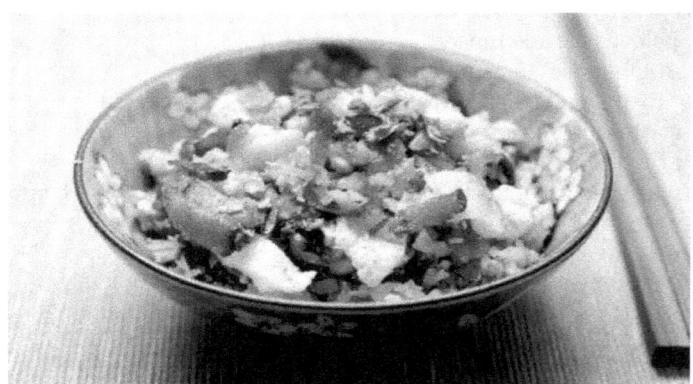

Ingredients

- 1 head of cauliflower
- ½ Vidalia onion
- 3 cloves of garlic
- 1 tbsp coconut oil
- salt and pepper, to taste
- This recipe makes 2-3 servings, depending on the size of your cauliflower.

Instructions

- Remove leaves and stem from cauliflower; discard. Grate the entire head of cauliflower until it resembles rice.
- Dice the onions and garlic to your desired size.
- Add coconut oil to a pan over medium heat. Add in onion and garlic until slightly browned.
- Add in grated cauliflower, salt, and pepper and stir until heated.

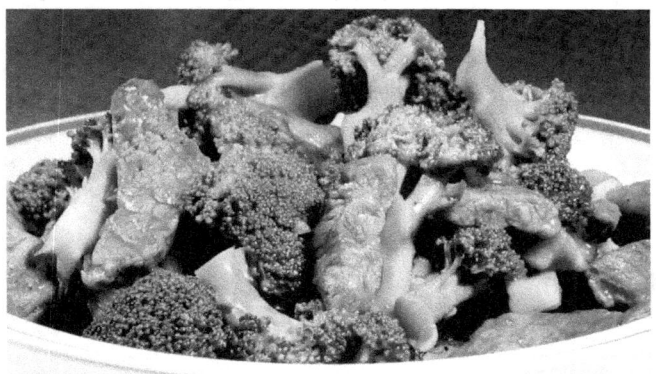

Ingredients

- 1.5 lbs. sirloin, thinly sliced
- 4 tbsp coconut aminos, divided
- 4 tbsp red wine vinegar, divided
- 3 tbsp chicken broth
- 4 cloves garlic, minced
- 1 tsp arrowroot flour
- 1 tsp honey
- 1 tbsp ginger, minced
- 1/2 tsp sesame oil
- 1 head broccoli, cut into florets
- 4 carrots, diagonally sliced
- 3 tbsp coconut oil, divided

Instructions

- Place the sirloin in a small bowl with one tablespoon each of red wine vinegar and coconut aminos and toss to coat. Let marinate for 15 minutes at room temperature.

- Meanwhile, whisk together 3 tablespoons each red wine vinegar, coconut aminos, and chicken broth. Stir in the garlic, ginger, arrowroot, honey, and sesame oil. Prepare a separate small bowl with 1 tablespoon of water and set it next to the stove along with the garlic sauce.
- Melt 2 tablespoons of coconut oil in a large skillet over medium heat. Place the steak in the skillet in a single layer. The meat should sizzle; otherwise the pan is not hot enough. Cook for 1-2 minutes per side to brown, and then transfer to a bowl.
- Add the remaining tablespoon of coconut oil to the skillet. Stir in the broccoli and carrots, cooking for 2 minutes. Add the water to the skillet and cover with a lid. Let cook for 2-3 minutes, then remove the lid and cook until all of the water has evaporated.
- Add the garlic mixture to the vegetables and stir to coat. Add the beef back into the pan and toss until the sauce thickens and everything is well coated. Serve immediately.

Notes

- Servings: 4-6
- Difficulty: Medium

Homemade Sweet and Salty Paleo Granola

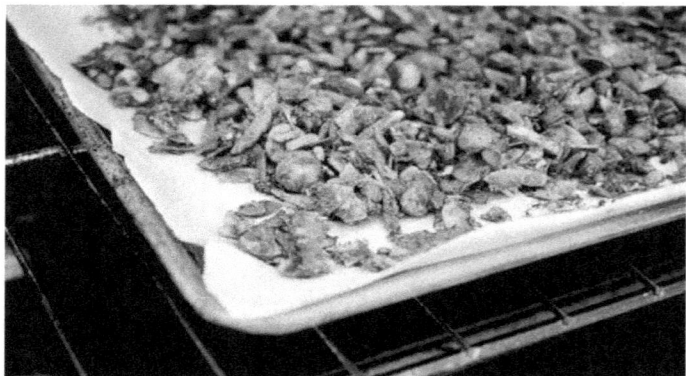

Ingredients

- 1 cup cashews
- 3/4 cup almonds
- 1/4 cup pumpkin seeds, shelled
- 1/4 cup sunflower seeds, shelled
- 1/2 cup unsweetened coconut flakes
- 1/4 cup coconut oil
- 1/4 cup honey
- 1 tsp vanilla
- 1 cup dried cranberries
- 1 tsp salt

Instructions

- Preheat oven to 300 degrees F. Line a baking sheet with parchment paper. Place the cashews, almonds, coconut flakes and pumpkin seeds into a blender and pulse to break the mixture into smaller pieces.
- In a large microwave-safe bowl, melt the coconut oil, vanilla, and honey together for 40-50 seconds. Add in the mixture from the blender and the sunflower seeds, and stir to coat.
- Spread the mixture out onto the baking sheet and cook for 20-25 minutes, stirring once, until the mixture is lightly browned. Remove from heat. Stir in the dried cranberries and salt.
- Press the granola mixture together to form a flat, even surface. Cool for about 15 minutes, and then break into chunks. Store in an airtight container or resealable bag.

Notes

- Servings: 6
- Difficulty: Easy

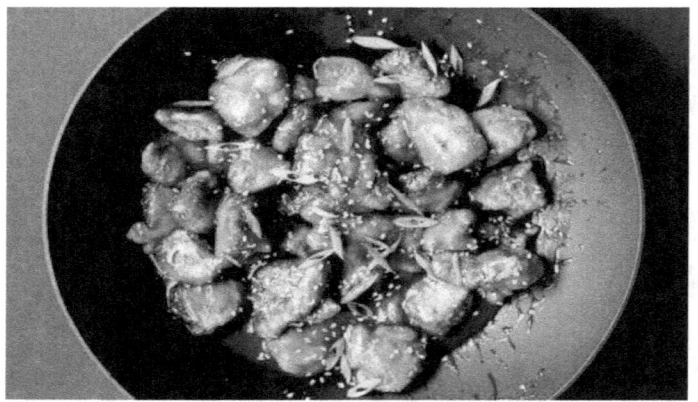

Ingredients

- 3 lbs. boneless beef roast, trimmed of fat
- 1 tbsp coconut oil
- 1 cup beef stock
- 5 carrots, peeled and diced
- 2 stalks celery, diced
- 1/2 large onion, sliced
- 3 garlic cloves, chopped
- 1 tbsp fresh parsley, chopped

For the spice rub

- 1 tbsp freshly ground black pepper
- 1 tbsp ground coriander
- 2 tsp cinnamon
- 1 1/2 tsp salt
- 1/2 tsp ground clove
- 1/2 tsp ground allspice

Instructions

- Mix together the ingredients for the spice rub and massage into the roast. Heat the coconut oil in a large skillet over medium-high heat. Add the roast to the pan and let sear for 5 minutes. Flip and repeat with the other side. Transfer the roast to the slow cooker.
- Add the carrots, onion, garlic, and celery to the slow cooker. Pour in the broth. Turn the heat on to low and cook for 6-7 hours, until the meat is tender. Serve hot sprinkled with chopped parsley.

Notes

- Servings: 6
- Difficulty: Easy

Hearty Paleo Jambalaya (Try This!)

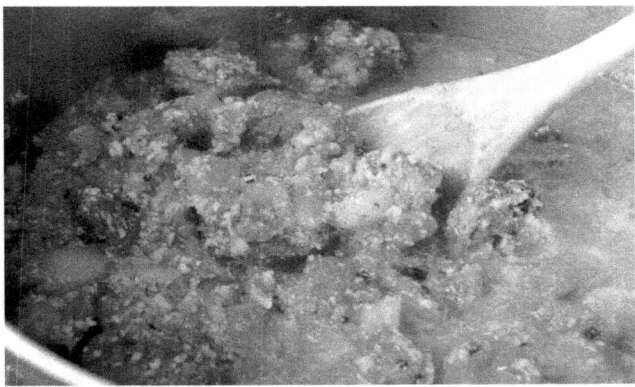

Ingredients

- 1 tbsp extra virgin olive oil
- 8 oz. Andouille sausage, diced
- 1/2 red bell pepper, diced
- 1/2 yellow bell pepper, diced
- 4 cloves garlic, minced
- 1/2 medium onion, diced

- 1 14.5-oz. can fire-roasted tomatoes
- 1 tbsp smoked paprika
- 1 tsp dried thyme
- 1 tsp cumin
- Dash of cayenne pepper
- 1 1/2 cups chicken broth
- 1 large head of cauliflower, coarsely chopped
- 1 lb. medium shrimp, peeled and deveined
- Salt and pepper, to taste
- Fresh cilantro, for garnish

Instructions

- Heat the olive oil in a Dutch oven or heavy-bottomed saucepan. Add the Andouille sausages and cook for 4-5 minutes until lightly browned. Add the red and yellow peppers, garlic, and onion and stir. Cook for 4 minutes until softened.
- Stir in the tomatoes and spices. Pour in the chicken stock and bring to a boil. Once boiling, turn the heat down and simmer for 20 minutes.
- Meanwhile, place the cauliflower into a food processor and pulse until it is reduced to the size of rice grains.
- Mix in the cauliflower rice to the jambalaya, starting with half of the rice and adding more depending on preference. Simmer for 12-15 minutes until tender. Add the shrimp and cook everything for 5-7 minutes until the shrimp are opaque. Season to taste with salt and pepper. Serve hot, garnished with fresh cilantro.

Notes

- Servings: 4-6
- Difficulty: Easy

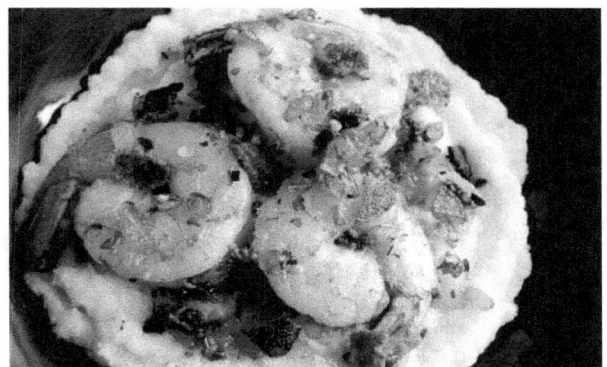

For the shrimp

- 15 pieces raw shrimp, shelled and de-veined
- 3 tbsp extra virgin olive oil
- 6 garlic cloves minced, divided
- Zest from one lemon
- 2 tsp dried oregano, divided
- 2 slices bacon
- 1/2 large onion, diced
- 2 tbsp butter
- 1 tbsp white wine vinegar
- 1 tsp red pepper flakes
- 1 tbsp lemon juice
- 1 tbsp chopped fresh oregano
- Salt and freshly ground black pepper, to taste

For the grits

- 1 large head of cauliflower, cut into florets
- 1/4 cup almond milk

- 4 garlic cloves, minced
- 1 tbsp ghee or butter
- 1/4 tsp cayenne pepper
- Salt and pepper, to taste

Instructions

- In a medium bowl mix together the olive oil, 2 cloves of garlic, lemon zest, and 1 teaspoon dried oregano. Place shrimp in the bowl and marinate for 1-3 hours.
- Place a couple inches of water in a large pot. Once water is boiling, place steamer insert and then cauliflower florets into the pot and cover. Steam for 12-14 minutes, until completely tender. Drain and return cauliflower to pot.
- Add the milk, ghee, and garlic to the cauliflower. Using an immersion blender, combine ingredients. The cauliflower should be fairly thick to resemble the consistency of grits. Season with salt and pepper to taste.
- Cook the bacon in a large skillet over medium heat until crispy. Reserving the bacon fat in the pan, set the bacon aside to cool and break into pieces.
- Add the butter to the bacon fat in the pan and melt. Add the onion and sauté for 4-5 minutes until softened. Add in the remaining 4 garlic cloves, dried oregano, and the red pepper flakes. Sauté for 1-2 minutes, stirring frequently.
- Stir in the white wine vinegar, and then add the shrimp. Cook, stirring frequently, until the shrimp are cooked through, 3-4 minutes. Remove from heat and stir in the lemon juice. Season with salt and pepper. Serve shrimp and onions over grits, with bacon and fresh oregano for garnish.

Notes

- Servings: 3-4
- Difficulty: Medium

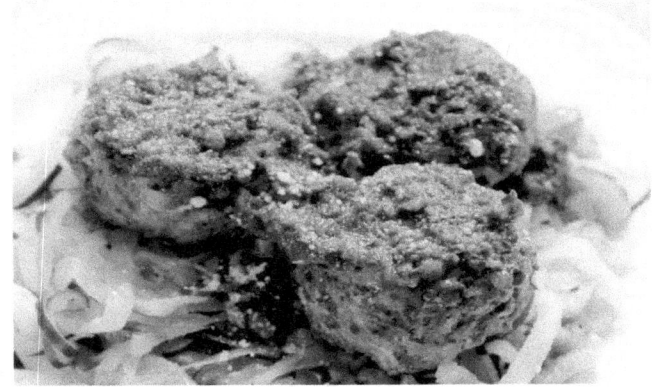

Ingredients

- 2 lbs. ground turkey
- 1/2 cup almond flour
- 1/2 cup pesto
- 2 egg whites
- 1/2 tsp salt
- 1/4 tsp freshly ground pepper

Instructions

- Preheat the oven to 375 degrees F. Line a baking sheet with aluminum foil and then place a wire cooling rack on top of the baking sheet. Coat the wire rack well with coconut oil spray.
- In a large bowl, mix together all of the ingredients. Roll the mixture into small balls using your hands and place on the wire rack. Bake for 20-25 minutes until cooked through.

Notes

- Servings: 24 meatballs
- Difficulty: Easy

DESSERTS

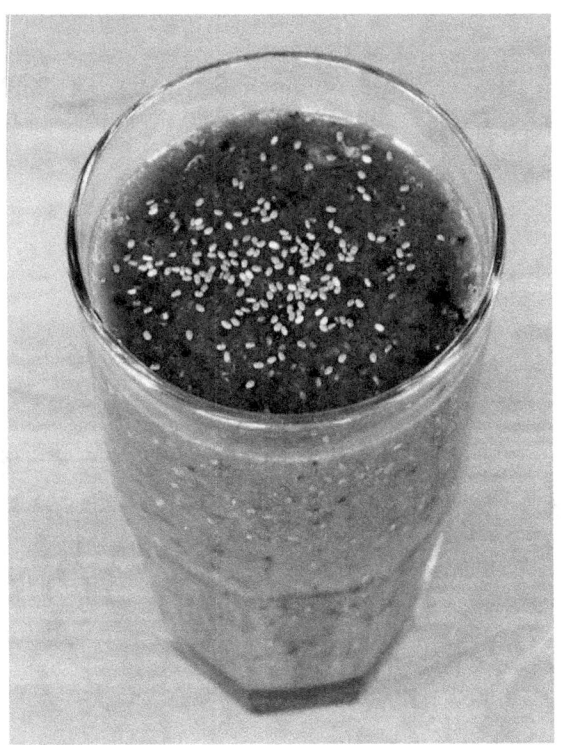

Ingredients

- 1/2 cup coconut milk
- 1/4 cup cold water
- 1/2 frozen banana

- 1/2 cup frozen raspberries
- 1/2 cup frozen blueberries
- 1 tbsp chia seeds

Directions

- In a large cup (if using an immersion blender) or a blender, combine ingredients and blend until smooth. Add more water if necessary to reach desired consistency. Serve immediately.

Notes

- Servings: 1
- Difficulty: Easy

Balsamic Green Bean Salad

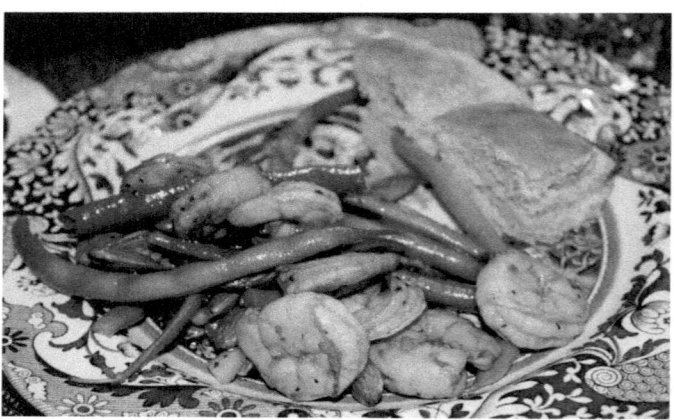

Ingredients

- 1 1/2 lbs green beans, trimmed and cut to 3 inch long pieces
- 1/2 red onion, finely chopped
- 3 tbsp olive oil
- 2 tbsp balsamic vinegar
- 1/3 cup chopped walnuts
- Salt and pepper to taste

Instructions

- Bring a pot of salted water to a boil. Add the green beans and blanch for 2-3 minutes. The beans should be just barely cooked through and still crisp. Prepare a large bowl of ice water while the beans are cooking. Remove beans from hot water and place into ice bath to stop the cooking. Drain.
- Place the green beans and red onion in a large bowl. Toss in the olive oil to coat. Sprinkle in the balsamic and season with salt and freshly ground black pepper. Top with chopped walnuts to serve.

Chocolate Bavarian Cheesecake

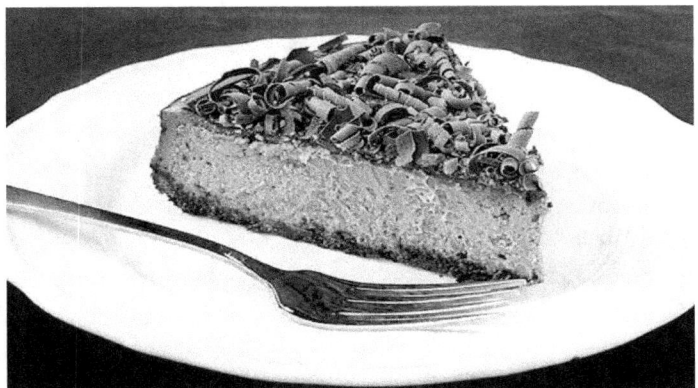

Ingredients:

<u>For the base:</u>

- 15 Easy Chocolate Cookies
- ¼ cup coconut oil (melted)

OR

- 2 cups nuts

- 1 cup dried dates (soaked in water)

<u>For the middle:</u>

- 2+1/2 cups raw cashews (soaked in water for 6 or more hours)
- ½ cup honey
- ¼ cup coconut oil
- ¼ cup cacao powder

- ½ cup coconut milk

- ½ cup orange juice

<u>For the top:</u>

- 1 can coconut cream (chilled in fridge overnight)
- Cacao nibs to decorate

Instructions:

<u>For the base:</u>

- Grind the chocolate cookies in a food processor until fine. Add the melted coconut oil and process until mixture sticks together. Add another tablespoon of coconut oil if you need to.

  Press the crumbs into the base of a 21cm springform tin. If you don't have a springform tin, just line your tin with plastic wrap or baking paper so you can remove it easily.

OR

- If you can't be bothered making the cookies (or didn't have any in the freezer like I did), just process 2 cups of nuts in a food processor until finely chopped. (Any combination of nuts works well. I've tried just macadamias and it is beautiful and also a combination of cashews, macadamias, hazelnuts, walnuts and brazil nuts)
- When your nuts are finely chopped, drain the soaked dates, getting out as much water as you can. Then add them to the food processor and process until it makes a sticky dough.
- Next, scoop the date & nut mixture into your pan. Put small plastic freezer bags onto your hands and use your fingers to spread the mixture evenly into the pan. (No sticky fingers!)

<u>For the filling:</u>

- Drain the cashews well. Put all of the filling ingredients into a high speed blender or processor and process until smooth. I have a new Froothie blender that is amazing! I compared it to the Vita Mix and it's cheaper and more powerful. You know I love a bargain. Anyway, I'm really happy with it and it makes amazing cheesecake filling!

- You will need to use the tamper if you have one and regularly scrape down the sides to make sure all the ingredients are blended together. Keep processing until it is super smooth. Lots of taste testing needed for this step!

- Once the mixture is smooth, scrape it all into your pan, on top of the base mixture. Spread it out with a spatula.

- Cover with plastic wrap, then put into the freezer for at least 6 hours to set.

- When ready to serve, take it from the freezer and defrost for around 30 minutes to soften slightly before cutting. (15 mins for minis.)
- While it's defrosting, beat the cream that rises to the top of the coconut cream after it's been refrigerated. Use electric beaters and add some honey to taste if you like.
- Spread or pipe the cream over the top of your cheesecake and decorate with cacao nibs.

Raw Brownie Bites

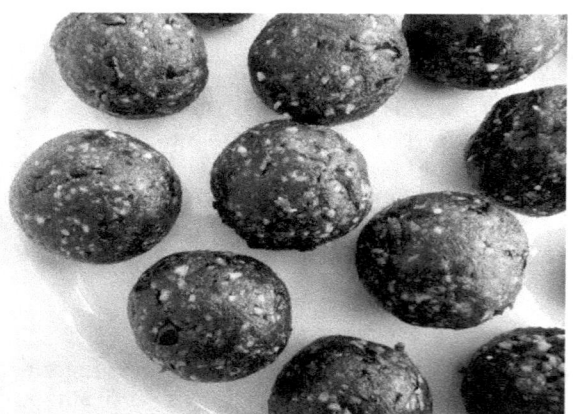

Ingredients

- 1 1/2 cups walnuts
- Pinch of salt
- 1 cup pitted dates
- 1 tsp vanilla
- 1/3 cup unsweetened cocoa powder

Instructions

- Add walnuts and salt to a blender or food processor. Mix until the walnuts are finely ground.
- Add the dates, vanilla, and cocoa powder to the blender. Mix well until everything is combined. With the blender still running, add a couple drops of water at a time to make the mixture stick together.
- Using a spatula, transfer the mixture into a bowl. Using your hands, form small round balls, rolling in your palm. Store in an airtight container in the refrigerator for up to a week.

Faux Paleo Napoleon

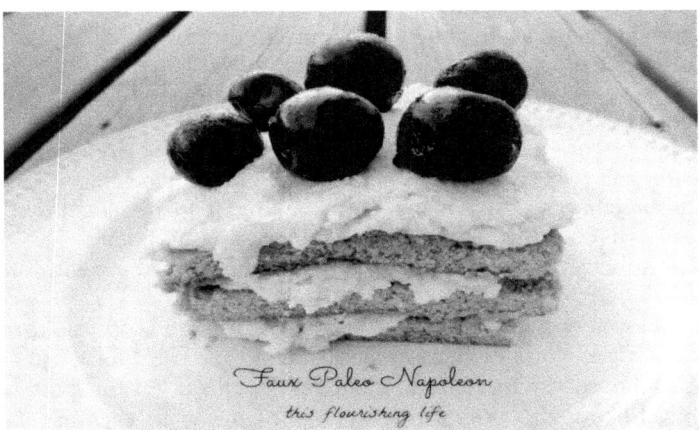

Faux Paleo Napoleon
this flourishing life

<u>Ingredients:</u>
Dough:
- 2 ½ cups almond flour
- ½ teaspoon baking soda
- ¼ teaspoon sea salt
- ½ cup + 2 tablespoons organic palm shortening, slightly melted so that it's easy to mix
- 2 tablespoons honey

- 1 tablespoon vanilla extract
- *Filling:*
- 2 cups almond flour
- ½ cup organic palm shortening or butter (I used shortening. Can't vouch for the results if butter is used, but I don't see why it wouldn't work.)
- ¼ cup honey
- 1 tablespoon vanilla extract
- ⅛ teaspoon sea salt
- 1 cup chopped fruit of choice for topping

Instruction:

- Preheat oven to 325 degrees.
- Mix all of the dry dough ingredients in a large bowl. Then add in all of the wet dough ingredients. Stir to combine.
- Move dough to a silicone baking mat or parchment paper, and roll it out with a rolling pin or something similar. If you need to use your hands, make sure you wet them with water first so that the dough doesn't stick to you.
- Using a pastry cutter, cut the dough into 12 equal-sized squares (or rectangles) about 3 (or 2.5) inches wide and 3 inches tall. No need to pull them apart. Once they're done baking, if you can't get them apart easily, just use the pastry cutter again to separate them.
- Carefully transfer the baking mat or parchment paper (with the dough on it) to a baking sheet.
- Bake for about 10-15 minutes, or until the dough is cooked through and a little bit crispy (like a pie crust would be).
- Mix all of the filling ingredients together, except for the fruit.
- Once the dough has cooled you can put your layers together. Layer a piece of dough, about 3-4 tablespoons of filling (spread it out), a piece of dough, more filling, a piece of dough, more filling, then some cherries.
- Begin a new one. Do this until you run out of dough and filling.
  - See more at: http://www.thisflourishinglife.com/2013/11/faux-paleo-napoleon-recipe.html#sthash.ubBMwq4b.dpuf

Homemade Strawberry Fruit Leather

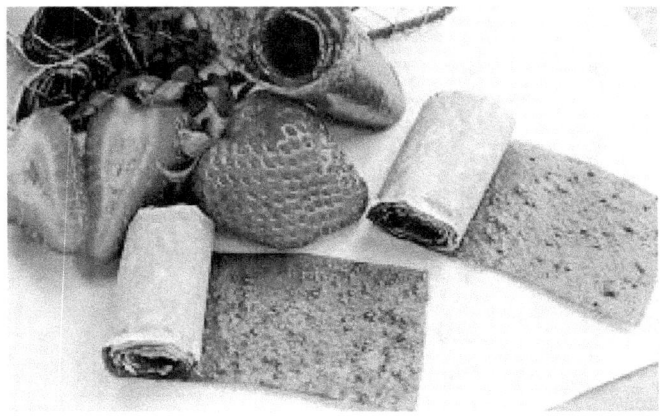

Ingredients

- 4 cups strawberries, hulled and chopped
- 2 tbsp honey

Instructions

- Preheat the oven to 170 degrees F or the lowest oven temperature setting. Line a baking sheet with a Silpat mat. Place strawberries in a medium saucepan and cook on low heat until soft. Add in the honey and stir to combine.
- Use an immersion blender to puree the strawberries in the saucepan, or transfer to a blender and puree until smooth. Pour the mixture onto the Silpat-lined baking sheet and spread evenly with a spatula. Bake for 6-7 hours, until it peels away from the parchment.
- Once cooled, peel the fruit leather off the mat and use a scissors to cut the fruit leather into strips. Roll up to serve, and store in an airtight container.

Notes

- Servings: approximately 12 strips
- Difficulty: Medium

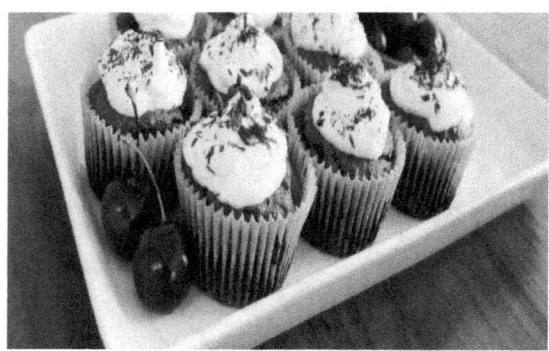

For the cupcakes

- 1/2 cup coconut flour
- 1/2 tsp baking powder
- 1/4 tsp salt
- 4 eggs
- 1/3 cup maple syrup
- 1/3 cup coconut oil, melted
- 2 tbsp almond milk
- 1 1/2 tsp vanilla extract

For the chocolate ganache

- 4 oz. dark chocolate
- 1/3 cup full-fat coconut milk, refrigerated

For the cupcakes

- Preheat the oven to 350 degrees F. Line a muffin tin with 8 cups and spray the insides with coconut oil spray to prevent sticking.
- Whisk together the coconut flour, baking powder, and salt in a large bowl. Add in the remaining ingredients and whisk until completely combined.

- Pour the batter into the muffin cups, dividing equally. Bake for 17-20 minutes, until a toothpick inserted into the center comes out clean. Place the muffin tin on a cooling rack and allow to cool for 10 minutes. Remove the cupcakes from the tin and cool completely before adding ganache.

For the chocolate ganache

- Melt the chocolate in the microwave, stirring regularly.
- Scoop the cream off the top of a can of chilled coconut milk. Combine with the chocolate and blend well. Let cool to room temperature before frosting cupcakes.

Notes

- Servings: 8
- Difficulty: Medium

Easy Homemade Gluten-Free Energy Bars

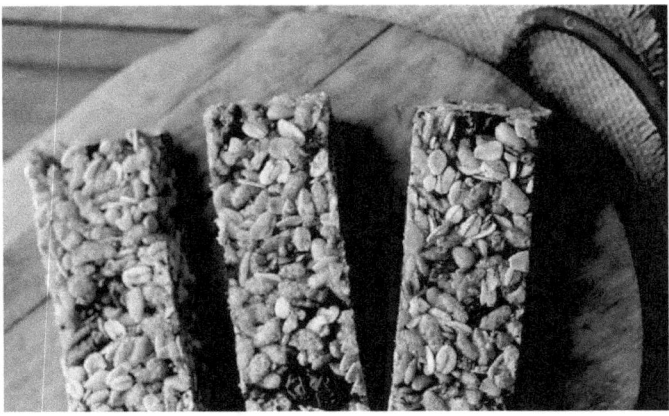

Ingredients

- 1 cup almonds

- 1 cup dried cranberries
- 1 cup pitted dates
- 1 tbsp unsweetened coconut flakes
- 1/4 cup mini dark chocolate chips

Instructions

- Combine all of the ingredients in a blender or food processor. Pulse a few times to break everything up. Then blend continuously until the ingredients have broken down and start to clump together into a ball.
- Using a spatula to scrape down the sides, turn out the mixture onto a piece of wax paper or plastic wrap. Press into an even square and chill, wrapped, for at least an hour. Cut into desired size of bars, wrapping each bar in plastic wrap to store in the fridge.

Notes

- Servings: 8 bars
- Difficulty: Easy

Coconut Macaroons with Chocolate and Pistachio

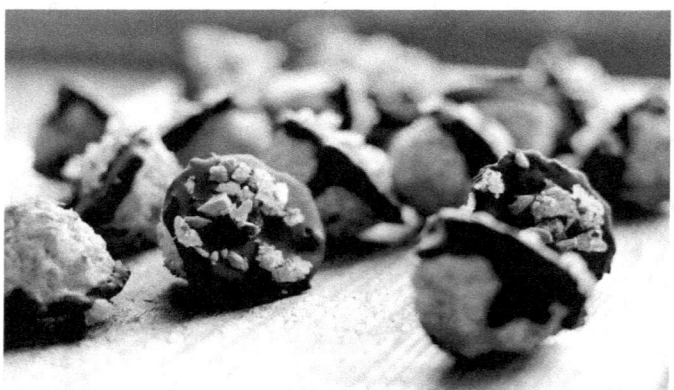

Ingredients

- 2 egg whites
- 1/4 cup honey
- 1 tsp vanilla extract
- Zest from 1 lemon
- Pinch of salt
- 1 1/2 cups grated coconut
- 2 tbsp ghee, melted

Coating

- 3 1/2 oz. dark chocolate
- 1 tsp coconut oil
- 1 tbsp pistachio nuts, shells removed

Instructions

- Preheat the oven to 350 degrees F. Line a baking sheet with parchment paper. In a large bowl, whisk together the egg whites, honey, vanilla, lemon zest, and salt until foamy. Mix in the ghee and coconut flakes. Let rest for 20 minutes to allow the coconut to soak up the liquid.
- Spoon 1 tightly packed tablespoon of the mixture onto the lined baking sheet. Repeat with remaining batter, and then bake for 8-12 minutes. Remove from the oven once the macaroons turn golden. Carefully transfer to a wire rack to cool completely.
- Finely chop the pistachio nuts and set aside. Prepare a double broiler and melt the chocolate and coconut oil for the coating. Dip the bottom of each macaroon in the chocolate and place on the wire rack with the chocolate side up. Sprinkle with chopped pistachios and allow to dry.

Notes

- Servings: about 20 small macaroons
- Difficulty: Medium

The Best Paleo Brownies (Chocolaty Goodness)

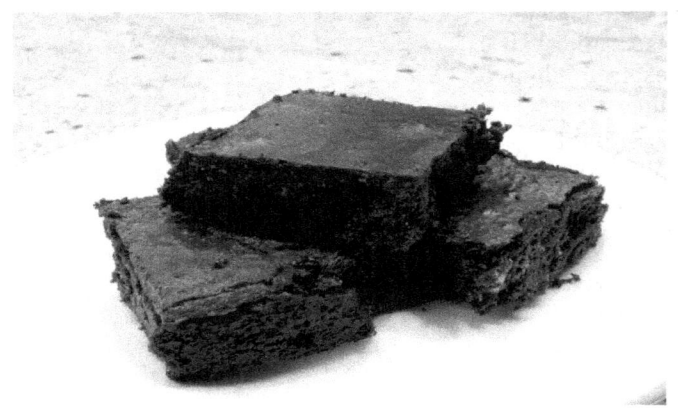

Ingredients

- 1 cup paleo-friendly almond butter
- 1/3 cup maple syrup
- 1 egg
- 2 tbsp ghee
- 1 tsp vanilla
- 1/3 cup cocoa powder
- 1/2 tsp baking soda

Instructions

- Preheat the oven to 325 degrees F. In a large bowl, whisk together the almond butter, syrup, egg, ghee, and vanilla. Stir in the cocoa powder and baking soda.
- Pour the batter into a 9-inch baking pan. Bake for 20-23 minutes, until the brownie is done, but still soft in the middle.

Notes

- Servings: 6
- Difficulty: Easy

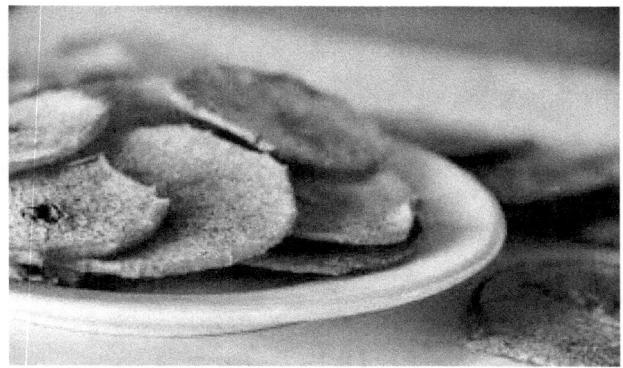

Ingredients

- 1-2 apples (I used Honeycrisp)
- 1 tsp cinnamon

Instructions

- Preheat oven to 200 degrees.
- Using a sharp knife or mandolin, slice apples thinly. Discard seeds. Prepare a baking sheet with parchment paper and arrange apple slices on it without overlapping. Sprinkle cinnamon over apples.
- Bake for approximately 1 hour, then flip. Continue baking for 1-2 hours, flipping occasionally, until the apple slices are no longer moist. Store in airtight container.

Paleo Pumpkin Pie Smoothie

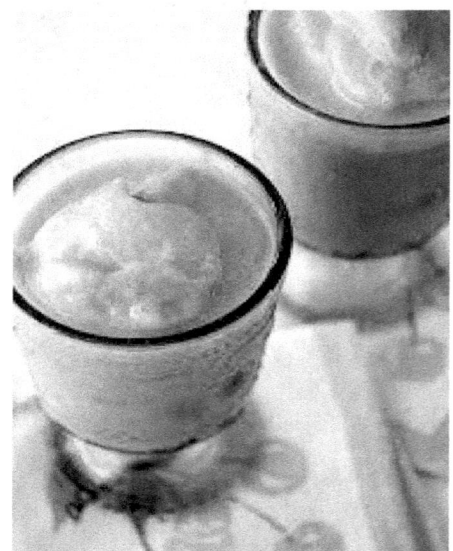

Ingredients

- 1 frozen banana
- 2 tbsp pumpkin puree
- ½ cup unsweetened almond milk
- ½ tsp vanilla extract
- 1 tsp honey
- 1 tbsp hemp hearts
- ¼ tsp cinnamon

- ¼ tsp cloves
- ¼ tsp nutmeg

Instructions

- Combine all ingredients in a blender and process until smooth. I find it's easier on the blender if I break the frozen banana into smaller chunks before processing.
- Pour into a tall glass and enjoy with your favorite book, your favorite music, or both!

Notes

- Calories: 220
- Total Fat: 6.4g
- Saturated Fat: 0.8g
- Carbs: 38.0g
- Fiber: 6.1g
- Protein: 5.6g

The Best Homemade Ranch Dressing Ever

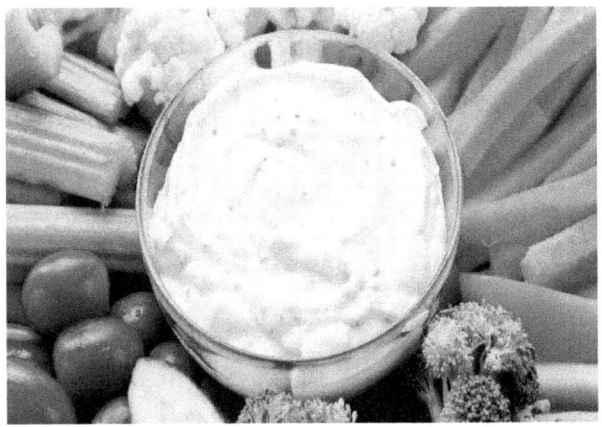

Ingredients

- 1/2 cup Paleo mayo (see below)
- 1/2 cup coconut milk
- 1/2 tsp onion powder
- 1 tsp garlic powder
- 1 tsp dill
- Salt and freshly ground pepper, to taste

Instructions

- Whisk all ingredients together to combine. Season with salt and pepper to taste. Store in an airtight container in the refrigerator for up to a week.

Mayo recipe

- 1 egg, room temperature
- 2 tbsp lemon juice or apple cider vinegar
- 1/2 tsp salt
- 1/2 tsp dry mustard
- 1 cup light olive oil*
- In a tall glass (if using an immersion blender) or a blender, place the egg and lemon juice. Let come to room temperature, about one hour. Add the salt and mustard. Blend ingredients. While blending, very slowly pour in the olive oil. Blend until it reaches desired consistency. Store in the refrigerator for up to a week.
- *It's important to use a light olive oil, not full flavor, for mayonnaise. You could also use almond or walnut oil instead.

Paleo Chocolate Cookies (I Can't Get Enough of These)

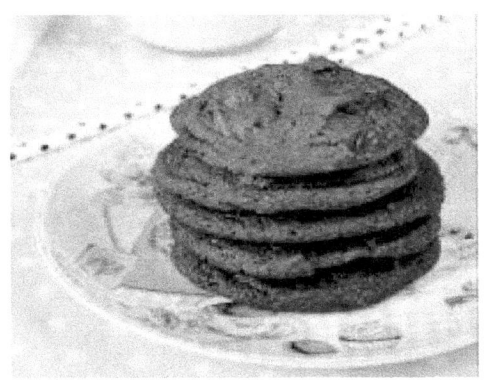

Ingredients

- 2 tbsp and 2 tsp coconut oil
- 3 oz. unsweetened dark chocolate
- 1/4 cup honey
- 2 eggs
- 1 1/2 tsp vanilla extract
- 1/2 cup coconut flour
- 1/2 tsp cinnamon

Instructions

- In a large microwave-safe bowl, melt the coconut oil and chocolate in the microwave, stirring intermittently. Let cool for 5 minutes.

- Add the eggs, vanilla, and honey to the chocolate mixture. Stir well to make sure not to scramble the eggs. Add in the coconut flour and cinnamon and mix well. Place in the refrigerator for approximately 30 minutes, until slightly hardened.
- Preheat oven to 350 degrees F. Roll out the dough between two pieces of parchment paper until 1/4-inch thick. Cut out shapes with a cookie cutter and carefully place on a parchment-lined baking sheet. Repeat this step for remaining dough.
- Bake cookies for 12-15 minutes. Allow to cool before serving.

Notes

- Servings: approximately 18 cookies
- Difficulty: Medium

Paleo French Toast with Blueberry Syrup

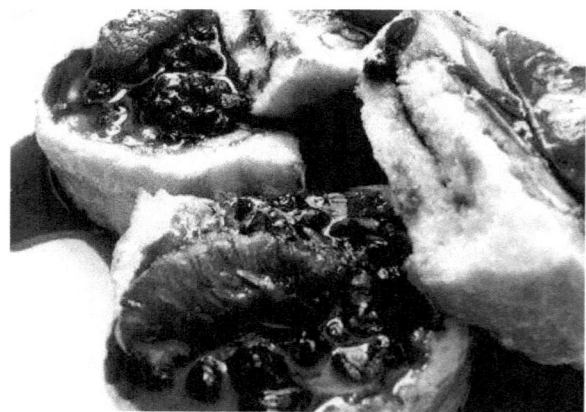

Ingredients

- 1 loaf Paleo bread (I used this recipe for Paleo Bread)
- 1/2 cup almond milk
- 2 eggs
- 1/2 tbsp vanilla
- 1 tsp cinnamon

Instructions

- In a large bowl, whisk together the coconut milk, eggs, vanilla and cinnamon.
- Heat a griddle or non-stick skillet to medium-high. Coat pan with coconut oil. Dip a slice of bread into the batter mixture to coat both sides, letting any excess drip off. Place the bread onto the pan and cook each side until slightly browned. Repeat with remaining bread. Serve warm.

Notes

- Servings: 4
- Difficulty: Easy

Lavender Maca Brownies (Dairy & Grain Free)

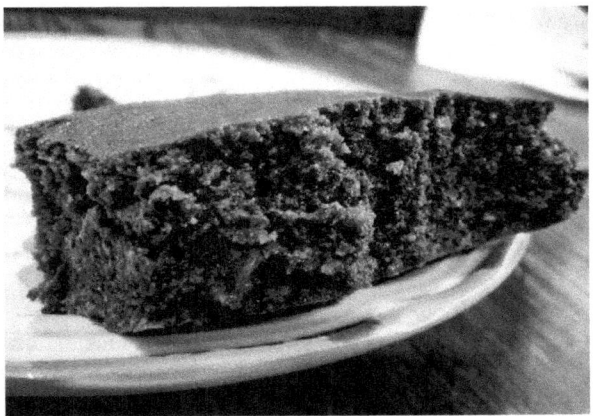

Ingredients

- 1/3 cup water
- 1/3 cup extra virgin olive oil
- 2 eggs
- 1 ½ cups almond flour
- 1 teaspoon baking powder
- 1 teaspoon salt
- 2/3 cup unsweetened cocoa powder
- 1 cup honey (I like to use raw honey found at my local farmer's market)
- ¾ cup semisweet chocolate chips
- 1 tablespoon dried lavender flowers (having a few left over for decoration)
- 1 tablespoon maca powder
- Himalayan pink salt (optional)

Directions

- Preheat oven to 350 degrees F and grease a 9x13" baking pan. (Brownies made in this size pan will be about one inch thick once baked – if you want them fuller, use a smaller sized pan)
- Whisk together the water, olive oil, and eggs in a large bowl.
- Slowly whisk in the flour, baking powder, salt, honey, maca powder, and cocoa powder one ingredient at a time. If you're using raw honey and it's too thick to whisk in, melt it in the microwave for about 20 seconds before adding it to your batter.
- Once the batter is well blended, add in your lavender and chocolate chips. The measurement for the lavender is up to you – I found one tablespoon to be the perfect amount, but depending on how floral you want these brownies to be you could add more or less.
- Pour the batter into a baking pan and spread until it is in one even layer. Don't worry if the batter seems too thick, that's how it's supposed to be.
- Bake for about 20 minutes, until a toothpick inserted in the center comes out clean.

- Let cool, then sprinkle fresh lavender and Himalayan pink salt over the top before cutting.
- Enjoy the fruits of your labor!!

Notes

1. This recipe should make approximately 24 2x2" square brownies.

Green Kale Smoothie with Mango

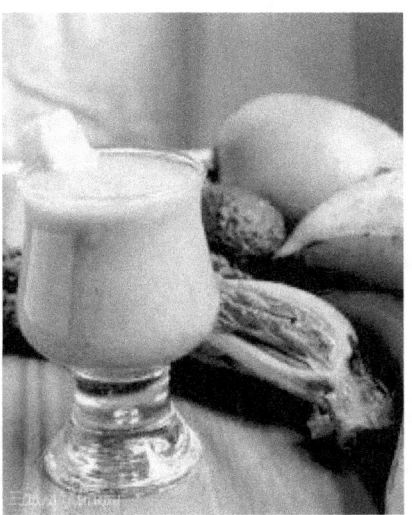

Ingredients

- 2 large leaves of kale

- 2 frozen bananas (peeled and cut into thirds)
- 1 frozen mango (diced)
- 2 tablespoons maca powder
- 2 tablespoons hemp hearts
- 3 cups unsweetened almond milk
- This recipe makes two large smoothies, can be halved for one serving.

Directions

- Add frozen banana chunks and frozen mango chunks into a blender with the almond milk. Blend until smooth. (I freeze my fruit in chunks to make it easier on the blender)
- Add in kale, maca powder, and hemp hearts. Blend until smooth.
- Serve immediately and enjoy!!

Nutrition Facts (per smoothie)

- Calories: 294
- Fat: 9.0g
- Saturated fat: 0.7g
- Sodium: 274mg
- Carbs: 51.0g
- Fiber: 8.6g
- Protein: 7.7g

Easy Paleo Shepherd's Pie

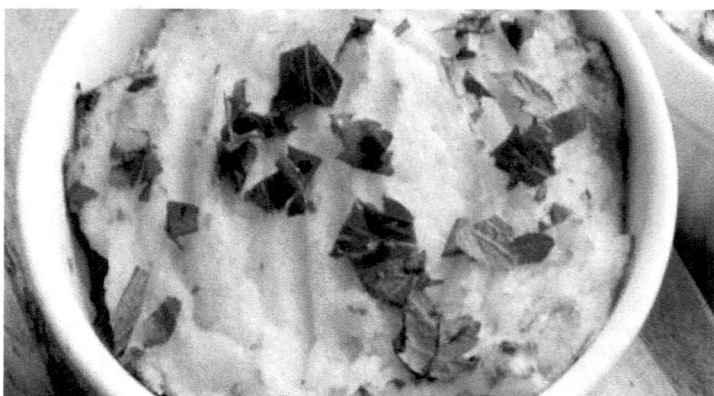

For the top layer

- 1 large head cauliflower, cut into florets
- 2 tbsp ghee, melted
- 1 tsp spicy Paleo mustard
- Salt and freshly ground black pepper, to taste
- Fresh parsley, to garnish

For the bottom layer

- 1 tbsp coconut oil
- 1/2 large onion, diced
- 3 carrots, diced
- 2 celery stalks, diced
- 1 lb. lean ground beef
- 2 tbsp tomato paste
- 1 cup chicken broth
- 1 tsp dry mustard
- 1/4 tsp cinnamon
- 1/8 tsp ground clove
- Salt and freshly ground black pepper, to taste

Instructions

- Place a couple inches of water in a large pot. Once the water is boiling, place steamer insert and then cauliflower florets into the pot and cover. Steam for 12-14 minutes, until tender. Drain and return cauliflower to the pot.
- Add the ghee, mustard, salt, and pepper to the cauliflower. Using an immersion blender or food processor, combine the ingredients until smooth. Set aside.
- Meanwhile, heat the coconut oil in a large skillet over medium heat. Add the onion, celery, and carrots and sauté for 5 minutes. Add in the ground beef and cook until browned.
- Stir the tomato paste, chicken broth, and remaining spices into the meat mixture. Season to taste with salt and pepper. Simmer until

most of the liquid has evaporated, about 8 minutes, stirring occasionally.

- Distribute the meat mixture evenly among four ramekins and spread the pureed cauliflower on top. Use a fork to create texture in the cauliflower and drizzle with olive oil. Place under the broiler for 5-7 minutes until the top turns golden. Sprinkle with fresh parsley and serve.

Notes

- Servings: 4
- Difficulty: Medium

Spicy Avocado Dill Dressing

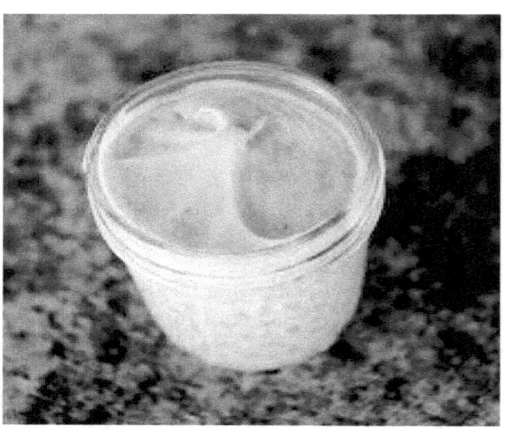

Ingredients

- 1 very ripe avocado
- 2 tablespoons olive oil
- 3 sprigs fresh dill

- 1 tbsp chili powder (more or less to taste)
- 1 tbsp lime juice
- 1 tbsp honey
- 2 tbsp apple cider vinegar
- 2 cloves garlic
- ¼ cup almond milk
- ¼ cup water

Directions

- Combine all ingredients in a blender, process until creamy.
- Store in an airtight jar or container in refrigerator, will last approximately 1 week.

Nutrition Facts per serving

- Calories: 104
- Fat: 9.2g
- Saturated Fat: 2.7g
- Carbs: 6.3g
- Fiber: 2.4g
- Protein: 1.1g

No-Bake Walnut Cookies (Grain-Free & Gluten-Free)

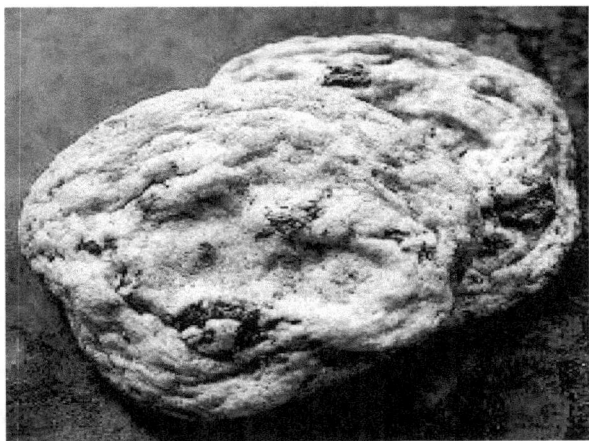

Ingredients

- 1 cup walnuts
- 1/2 cup unsweetened coconut flakes
- 2 tbsp raw honey
- 1/2 tsp vanilla extract
- 1/4 tsp salt

Directions

- Add walnuts to food processor and blend until finely ground. Add in the remaining ingredients and blend until a dough forms, about a minute.
- Turn out the dough onto a piece of parchment paper. Using your hands, roll pieces of the dough into small balls, about 1 inch around, and space out on parchment paper. After all of the balls are formed, press down on each ball to form a flat cookie. Place in the freezer for at least 30 minutes before serving. Store in an airtight container in the freezer.

Notes

- Servings: Makes 10-12 cookies
- Difficulty: Easy

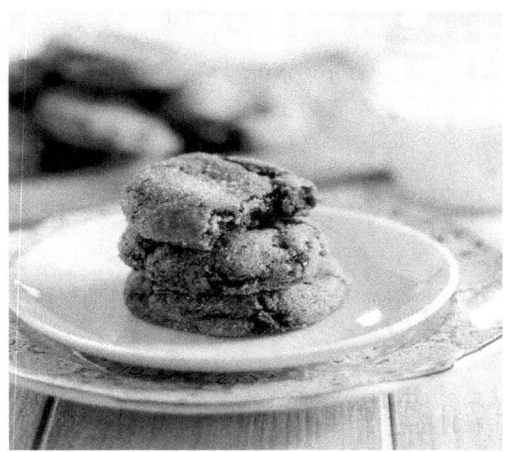

Ingredients

- 2 tbsp and 2 tsp coconut oil
- 3 oz. unsweetened dark chocolate
- 1/4 cup honey
- 2 eggs
- 1 1/2 tsp vanilla extract
- 1/2 cup coconut flour
- 1/2 tsp cinnamon

Instructions

- In a large microwave-safe bowl, melt the coconut oil and chocolate in the microwave, stirring intermittently. Let cool for 5 minutes.
- Add the eggs, vanilla, and honey to the chocolate mixture. Stir well to make sure not to scramble the eggs. Add in the coconut flour and cinnamon and mix well. Place in the refrigerator for approximately 30 minutes, until slightly hardened.
- Preheat oven to 350 degrees F. Roll out the dough between two pieces of parchment paper until 1/4-inch thick. Cut out shapes with a cookie

cutter and carefully place on a parchment-lined baking sheet. Repeat this step for remaining dough.
- Bake cookies for 12-15 minutes. Allow to cool before serving.

Notes

- Servings: approximately 18 cookies

- Difficulty: Medium

Paleo French Toast with Blueberry Syrup

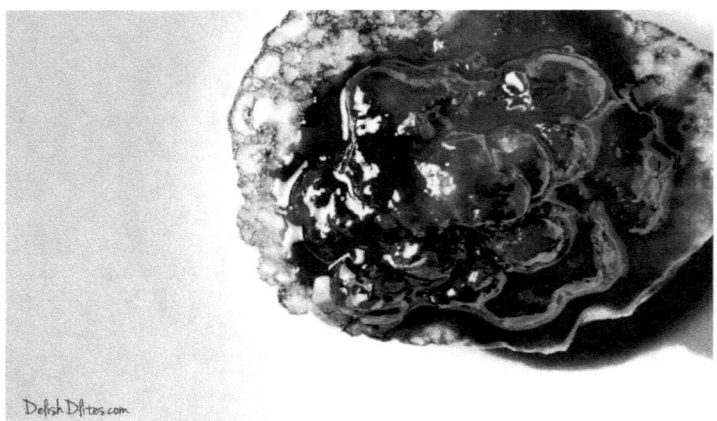

Delish Dlites.com

Ingredients

- 1 loaf Paleo bread (I used this recipe for Paleo Bread)
- 1/2 cup almond milk
- 2 eggs
- 1/2 tbsp vanilla
- 1 tsp cinnamon

Instructions

- In a large bowl, whisk together the coconut milk, eggs, vanilla and cinnamon.
- Heat a griddle or non-stick skillet to medium-high. Coat pan with coconut oil. Dip a slice of bread into the batter mixture to coat both sides, letting any excess drip off. Place the bread onto the pan and cook each side until slightly browned. Repeat with remaining bread. Serve warm.

Notes

- Servings: 4
- Difficulty: Easy

Lavender Maca Brownies (Dairy & Grain Free)

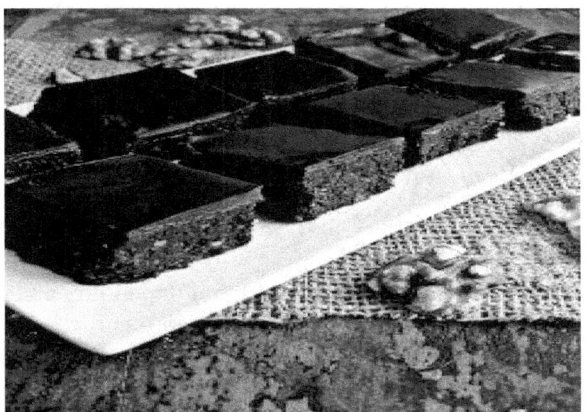

Ingredients

- 1/3 cup water
- 1/3 cup extra virgin olive oil
- 2 eggs
- 1 ½ cups almond flour
- 1 teaspoon baking powder

- 1 teaspoon salt
- 2/3 cup unsweetened cocoa powder
- 1 cup honey (I like to use raw honey found at my local farmer's market)
- ¾ cup semisweet chocolate chips
- 1 tablespoon dried lavender flowers (having a few left over for decoration)
- 1 tablespoon maca powder
- Himalayan pink salt (optional)

Directions

- Preheat oven to 350 degrees F and grease a 9x13" baking pan. (Brownies made in this size pan will be about one inch thick once baked – if you want them fuller, use a smaller sized pan)
- Whisk together the water, olive oil, and eggs in a large bowl.
- Slowly whisk in the flour, baking powder, salt, honey, maca powder, and cocoa powder one ingredient at a time. If you're using raw honey and it's too thick to whisk in, melt it in the microwave for about 20 seconds before adding it to your batter.
- Once the batter is well blended, add in your lavender and chocolate chips. The measurement for the lavender is up to you – I found one tablespoon to be the perfect amount, but depending on how floral you want these brownies to be you could add more or less.
- Pour the batter into a baking pan and spread until it is in one even layer. Don't worry if the batter seems too thick, that's how it's supposed to be.
- Bake for about 20 minutes, until a toothpick inserted in the center comes out clean.
- Let cool, then sprinkle fresh lavender and Himalayan pink salt over the top before cutting.
- Enjoy the fruits of your labor!!

Notes

This recipe should make approximately 24 2x2" square brownies.

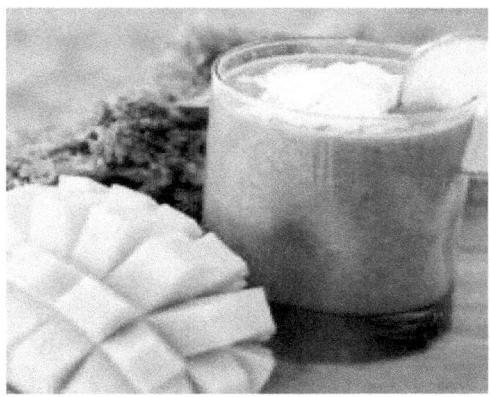

Ingredients

- 2 large leaves of kale
- 2 frozen bananas (peeled and cut into thirds)
- 1 frozen mango (diced)
- 2 tablespoons maca powder
- 2 tablespoons hemp hearts
- 3 cups unsweetened almond milk
- This recipe makes two large smoothies, can be halved for one serving.

Directions

- Add frozen banana chunks and frozen mango chunks into a blender with the almond milk. Blend until smooth. (I freeze my fruit in chunks to make it easier on the blender)
- Add in kale, maca powder, and hemp hearts. Blend until smooth.
- Serve immediately and enjoy!!

Nutrition Facts (per smoothie)

- Calories: 294
- Fat: 9.0g

- Saturated fat: 0.7g
- Sodium: 274mg
- Carbs: 51.0g
- Fiber: 8.6g
- Protein: 7.7g

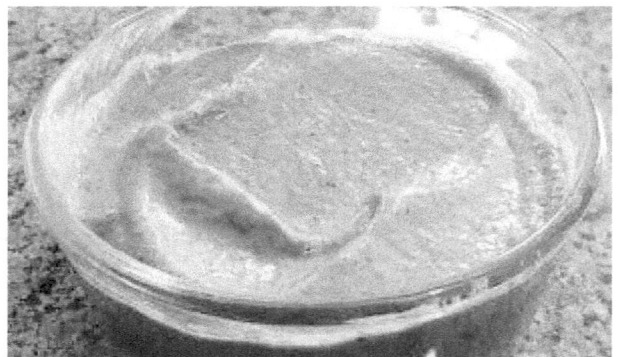

Ingredients

- 1 very ripe avocado
- 2 tablespoons olive oil
- 3 sprigs fresh dill
- 1 tbsp chili powder (more or less to taste)
- 1 tbsp lime juice
- 1 tbsp honey
- 2 tbsp apple cider vinegar
- 2 cloves garlic
- ¼ cup almond milk
- ¼ cup water

Directions

- Combine all ingredients in a blender, process until creamy.
- Store in an airtight jar or container in refrigerator, will last approximately 1 week.

Nutrition Facts per serving

- Calories: 104
- Fat: 9.2g
- Saturated Fat: 2.7g
- Carbs: 6.3g
- Fiber: 2.4g
- Protein: 1.1g

No-Bake Walnut Cookies (Grain-Free & Gluten-Free)

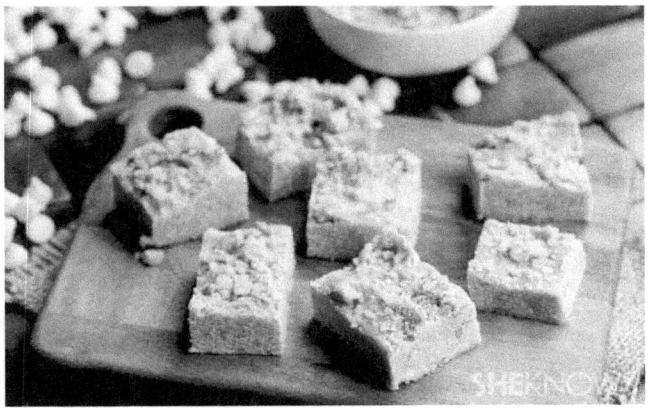

Ingredients

- 1 cup walnuts
- 1/2 cup unsweetened coconut flakes
- 2 tbsp raw honey
- 1/2 tsp vanilla extract

- 1/4 tsp salt

Directions

- Add walnuts to food processor and blend until finely ground. Add in the remaining ingredients and blend until a dough forms, about a minute.
- Turn out the dough onto a piece of parchment paper. Using your hands, roll pieces of the dough into small balls, about 1 inch around, and space out on parchment paper. After all of the balls are formed, press down on each ball to form a flat cookie. Place in the freezer for at least 30 minutes before serving. Store in an airtight container in the freezer.

Notes

- Servings: Makes 10-12 cookies
- Difficulty: Easy

Homemade Paleo Tortilla Chips

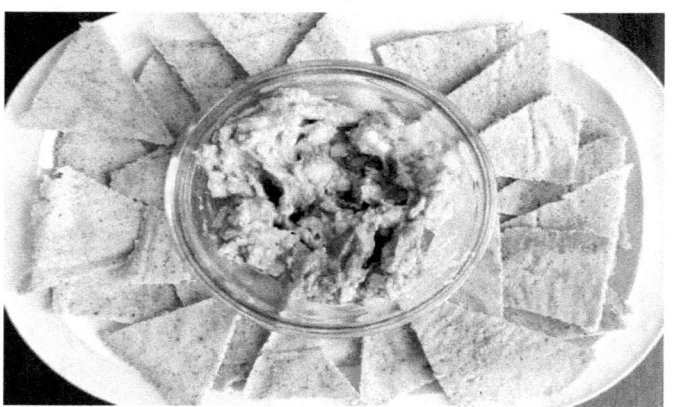

Ingredients

- 1 cup almond flour
- 1 egg white

- 1/2 tsp salt
- 1/2 tsp chili powder
- 1/2 tsp garlic powder
- 1/2 tsp cumin
- 1/4 tsp onion powder
- 1/4 tsp paprika

Directions

- Preheat the oven to 325 degrees F. In a large bowl, combine all of the ingredients together until they form an even dough.
- Roll out the dough between two pieces of parchment paper, as thinly as possible. Remove the top layer of parchment paper. Cut the dough into desired shapes for chips.
- Move the dough, with the parchment paper, onto a baking sheet. Bake for 11-13 minutes, until golden brown. Remove from the oven and let cool 5 minutes. Use a spatula to remove the chips from the paper. Serve with guacamole or salsa.

Refreshing Tomato Salsa Bowl Appetizer

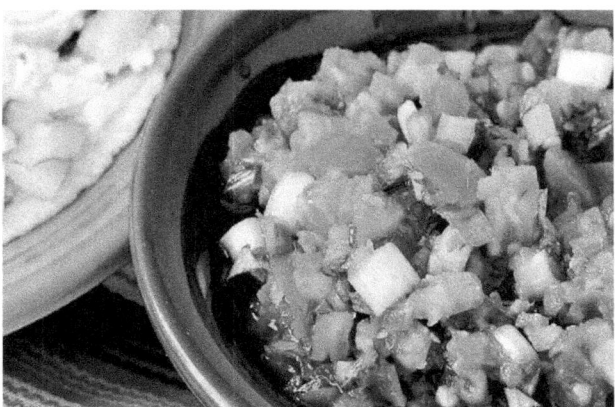

Ingredients

- 4 medium ripe Roma tomatoes
- 1/4 cup black olives, sliced
- 1/4 cup onion, finely diced
- 1/2 green bell pepper, seeded and chopped
- 1/2 jalapeno, seeded and finely chopped
- 2 cloves garlic, minced
- 1 tbsp fresh cilantro, chopped
- 1 tbsp grapeseed oil
- 2 tsp balsamic vinegar
- Salt and pepper, to taste

Instructions

- Slice the tomatoes in half and scoop out the insides. In a small bowl, mix together the remaining ingredients. Stir well. Spoon the salsa mixture into the tomato cups. Serve chilled.

Notes

- Servings: 4
- Difficulty: Easy

All-Natural Homemade Paleo Apple Butter

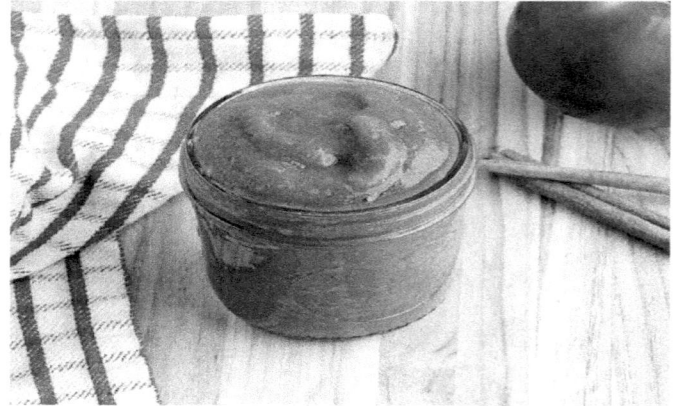

Ingredients

- 5 apples, peeled, cored and diced
- 2/3 cup apple cider
- 1/3 cup honey
- 1 tbsp cinnamon
- 1/2 tsp salt
- Pinch of cloves, optional

Instructions

- Place all of the ingredients into the slow cooker and stir to evenly coat. Cover and cook on low heat for 6 hours. Let cool slightly and puree in a food processor or blender until smooth.

Notes

- Servings: 4-6
- Difficulty: Easy

Herbed Calamari Salad with Preserved Lemons

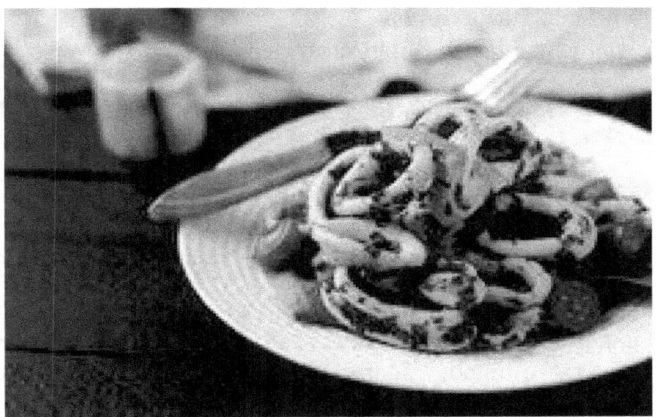

Ingredients

- 3 Tablespoons extra virgin olive oil
- 2 to 3 medium cloves garlic, smashed and minced
- 2 1/2 pounds cleaned and trimmed uncooked calamari rings and tentacles (defrosted)
- 3/4 teaspoon kosher salt
- 1/4 teaspoon freshly ground black pepper
- pinch crushed red pepper flakes
- juice of 1 large lemon
- 1/4 cup finely chopped mint leaves
- 1/4 cup finely chopped cilantro leaves
- 1/2 cup finely chopped flat-leaf parsley leaves
- peel of 1 preserved lemon, thinly sliced

Instructions

PREP:

- Begin by defrosting the calamari (if purchased frozen). Place in a strainer and run under cold water for 15 to 20 minutes, tossing a couple of times, until soft and pliable. Drain water, pat dry with paper towels and set aside.

- Use a paring knife to remove just the rind from the preserved lemon. Discard the inside and thinly slice the rind.

- Smash garlic and mince. Finely chop cleaned mint, cilantro and parsley.

COOK:

- Heat a very large skillet or frying pan over medium high heat. Once hot, add 1 1/2 Tablespoons of olive oil. Heat oil and add garlic.

- Saute, stirring constantly, for 20 to 30 seconds until fragrant and add in defrosted and well-drained calamari (If your pan isn't large enough to accommodate all the calamari in one layer, divide the 1 1/2 T olive oil and cook the calamari in batches. You do not want them to steam, you want them to sear and for that, they must cook in a single layer with some room around them).Sprinkle with a pinch of salt and pepper and continue cooking for 2 to 4 minutes or until opaque and just firm. You do not want to overcook the calamari or it be have a rubbery texture.

- Drain off any liquid that is released during cooking and remove cooked calamari to a mixing bowl.

- Add remaining 1 1/2 Tablespoons olive oil, salt, pepper, red pepper flakes, lemon juice, preserved lemon rind and herbs to mixing bowl and toss well while calamari still warm.

- Adjust seasoning if necessary, cover and chill until ready to serve. This is nice served over some spring greens or other delicate lettuce with some ripe cucumbers or grape tomatoes. Enjoy!

Healthy Fruit Leather

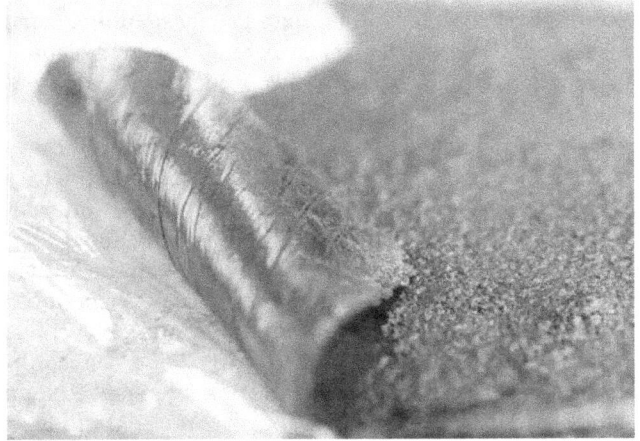

Ingredients

- 2 apples, finely diced
- 10 strawberries, diced
- 1 ruby pink grapefruit, diced
- Stevia/rice malt syrup to sweeten if needed
- 1 tsp cinnamon
- Pinch salt
- 1/4 cup water

Instructions

- Place the fruit in saucepan with the water and bring to a boil. Reduce the heat and simmer until the fruit is soft and the liquid has been reduced. Stir through the cinnamon and salt.
- Transfer the fruit to a blender and puree until smooth. Taste the mixture and if required add a sweetener. The grapefruit can be quite tart and while suitable for adults children may not appreciate this. If you would like a sweeter roll up than I suggest adding some sweetness to balance out the sourness. If a sweetener is added blend again until combined. You should end up with 2-3 cups worth of pureed fruit.
- Heat oven to 120-150°C (250-300F). Line a large baking tray with baking paper (if your baking tray is not very large you may need to use two smaller sized trays). Pour the mixture onto the tray and spread it out thinly by using the back of a spatula. You want it to just cover the baking paper's surface without leaving any gaps (the thinner the better!). Place the baking tray in the oven on the lowest shelf availiable and bake for 8-12 hours. I left mine overnight baking at about 130°C for 9 hours. Remove the tray from the oven and using a sharp knife cut the fruit leather into strips. Let it cool completely before peeling the fruit leather off the baking paper. Roll up if desired and store in an airtight container for up to a week! Enjoy :)

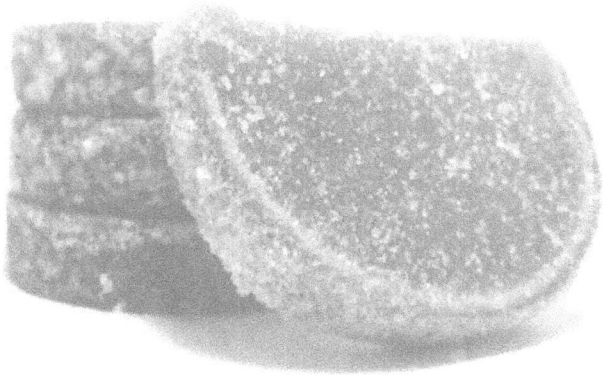

Ingredients:

- 1 T. vanilla extract
- ½ t. natural orange flavor
- Pinch real salt
- 1 ½ t. liquid stevia (every brand varies in sweetness, so add this 'to taste')
- 8 T. grassfed gelatin
- 1 can coconut milk
- 1 ½ C. water
- Natural orange food coloring to desired color
- orange ice cube tray molds

INSTRUCTIONS:

- Heat water and coconut milk over low heat until simmering.

- Continue on low heat, slowly adding in each tablespoon of gelatin, whisking the entire time.
- Add remaining ingredients and whisk until any clumps of gelatin are gone.
- Pour into molds, and pour remaining liquid into 8X8 glass pan.
- Put in fridge until solid. Gummis should pop out easily once hardened.

Thank you for downloading this book!

I hope this book was able to help you to be familiar with Paleo diet, the basic information about the diet regimen, and how you can obtain its healthy benefits. The "PALEO: The Healthy New You with Paleo" also contains a sample meal plan and great recipes that will serve as a starter during your transitioning to Paleo. More ultimately, this book includes unique Paleo recipes that you can try at home, and share with your loved ones.

The next step is to share your entire Paleo journey with your family and friends. The great benefits of the diet regimen may encourage them to try and change their current lifestyles. If that is the case, you can share all the knowledge you have learned in this book. Share some tips, cook recipes together and motivate each other while obtaining the benefits of doing Paleo.

Finally, If you enjoyed this book, I would really appreciate it if you could leave me a positive review on Amazon.

I love getting feedback from my customers, and reviews on Amazon really do make a difference. I read all of my reviews and would appreciate your thoughts.

Thanks so much.

Annabel Jacobs

www.ingramcontent.com/pod-product-compliance
Lightning Source LLC
Chambersburg PA
CBHW062148280526
45788CB00001B/348